BALANCE & STRENGTH TRAINING FOR SENIORS 101

SIMPLE HOME EXERCISES TO IMPROVE CORE STRENGTH, STABILITY AND POSTURE

VERNON FISHER

CONTENTS

INTRODUCTION

Don't let your age control your lifestyle, let your lifestyle control your age.

Danny sits on his porch and watches his neighbors on a sunny afternoon. He smiles at his neighbor helping his son learn to ride a bike on the sidewalk. He sees the boy's mom clapping and jumping on the porch. Across the street he sees a girl tying a kayak to the top of her car. He smiles as he watches a jogger go by, and waves at the mailman after he puts his mail in his mailbox.

As Danny goes to stand up, his wrist and knees pop. He feels that usual jolt of pain up his back when he goes from sitting to standing. He waits a few moments to let his blood pressure settle, before moving forward to the stairs on his front porch. As he reaches the top stair, he feels a little dizzy and realizes his cane is inside. He knows if he decides to go down the stairs without his cane, it could end badly. He leans against the post on his porch and looks back out at his neighbors and sighs. They laugh and bounce through the neighborhood. Tackling stairs and running around the yard as Danny tries to catch his breath. He sees his reflection in his front door and thinks to himself, "to be young again."

Growing old can be a beautiful thing. It's a journey of your life. It's natural. Being older means being able to look back on all the people you have touched in your life. You can see all the lessons you've learned and how much you've grown as a person. You get to relive all of your best accomplishments and smile at the memories you've made with friends and family.

Looking back on all the positives in your life can leave you wanting more from life. You can start to fear growing dependent on others or being unable to do what you love. Comparing yourself to your 30-year-old self can make you start a list of things you wish were different. Maybe you wish you could still run on the treadmill. Or chase your grandkids through the yard. Or plant some flowers without having knee and back pain.

You might feel sad or discouraged when you think about your health. If you have feelings of hopelessness, low self-esteem, or health issues that just seem to make your life harder, then you are in the right place.

Like Danny, we all experience issues and medical barriers. We get those familiar feelings of dread and desire to do something more. Exercise can be beneficial for people of all ages. Someone can exercise despite their age, location, equipment, health condition, or disability. The great thing about exercise is you don't have to run 10 miles a day to consider getting a workout in.

In this book, you'll learn about the aging process of your muscles and body. You'll learn quick, effective workouts for every part of the body. The exercises can be done with your body weight, so you don't even need equipment to make yourself healthier, happier, and more confident!

Throughout the book, you will explore ways to

- Decrease pain and discomfort associated with aging and older conditions.
- Strengthen your muscles.
- Improve mobility and joint movement.
- Benefit mental health.
- Build confidence.
- Get your life and independence back.

Despite your situation, exercise can be fun! It's important that you enjoy your workout. If you don't, how long would you stick with it? First, let's talk about what your goals are. Why did you pick up this book? What is one thing you wish you could change about your health? What are some common obstacles you encounter? Ask yourself these important questions so you know what you want to get out of exercising. Danny wanted to walk down the stairs on his front porch without a cane.

Deciding to start is the first step toward changing your life. This book covers exercising, in a step-by-step method, instructing those who don't even know where to start. *Wanting* to start, is all you need.

Choosing to start exercising will not only benefit you, but it will benefit the people in your life, as well. Your friends and family will notice the improvement in your health and mood. You may have to see your chiropractor, massage therapist, or physical therapist less. Your grandkids will be able to run around and play with you. You will act as an inspiration to all of those around you. Especially yourself.

Knowing what you want out of life will help you pick the exercises that are best for you. Some specific exercises can work on leg muscles and walking more steadily. Others can improve wrist and elbow movement, so you can knit and garden longer. There are exercises you can do to improve back pain and improve your core strength and balance.

Exercise can be beneficial in the short-term and long-term. Exercising, even just one time can momentarily improve mood and discomfort. Exercising in the long-term can improve strength and lead to more permanent improvements, like being able to walk farther, and longer.

The book will cover many different exercise combinations, perfect for anyone looking to better themselves and their health. These exercises can help prevent falls, which can lead to critical events. They also improve bone density, lessening the chance of broken bones.

Not only will exercise benefit current conditions, but it could keep some other conditions from forming or worsening. Exercise as a senior could improve heart and blood pressure issues, arthritis, decreased movement and mobility, mood disorders, mental distress, and the ability to perform activities of daily living (toileting, dressing, cooking, etc.).

Now that you know why you want to make yourself better, why it's important to work out, and what you can gain from exercising. The only thing to do now is have fun!

As always, check with a medical provider before beginning an exercise regimen.

1

WHY SHOULD YOU STRENGTH TRAIN AT 60+?

Regardless of age, strength training can help everyone. Whether you're 11 or 91, strength training can be beneficial for many reasons. Disabilities and health concerns may prevent a 91-year-old from doing exercises for an 11-year-old, but that doesn't mean the 91-year-old should hold back from strength training.

Normal aging processes in the body change the way we move and operate. As we get older:

Our metabolism slows down.

- Muscle mass and strength decrease
- Body fat increases.
- Bone density decreases.

- The small holes in our bones widen, making them weaker.
- Joints get stiff.
- Risk of falls and balance issues increase.
- The maximum amount of oxygen our body uses decreases.
- Reaction times and reflexes slow down.

These conditions, however, can be slowed, improved, and even sometimes reversed with strength training combined with a healthy diet and lifestyle.

BENEFITS

Strength training and exercise have immediate benefits, as well as long-term benefits. Short-term benefits are seen either right after exercise or in the following days. Long-term benefits can come from strength training and exercise regularly. Short-term benefits include making it easier to perform activities of daily living, reducing the chances of falls, and preventing some diseases.

Activities of daily living include going to the bathroom, putting on clothes, eating, etc. As we get older, activities of daily living can get harder for us to perform. Strength training allows older adults to be more independent, increase confidence, and develop a sense of purpose. Older adults who add strength training to their life have an easier time completing activities of daily living.

The risk of falls increases as we get older. Falls are so important in the older population because they can be very detrimental to health and well-being. Many older adults have a fear of falling from exercise. Strength training, however, will improve your balance and make you less likely to fall. Strength training also strengthens bones, so if you were to experience a fall, the chances of you breaking a bone are less than if you didn't exercise. Strength training also decreases the damage and problems associated with a fall.

Many diseases accumulate as we age, as well as an increased risk of developing other conditions and health problems. Conditions like diabetes, arthritis, heart disease, obesity, and osteoporosis can be prevented and even reversed through strength training. Some of the mental benefits of strength training include reducing stress, increasing happiness, and reducing the risk of Alzheimer's and dementia.

Exercise makes stress easier to handle, directly and indirectly. Senior adults can commonly experience anxiety and insomnia. Endorphins are released by exercise and can be used to improve sleep and anxiety. When you are stressed, you sleep poorly. When you sleep poorly, it is easier to become stressed.

One of the great short-term (and long-term) benefits of exercising is improved sleep. Our sleep can be affected by a number of reasons in our golden years. Strength training helps you sleep deeper, longer, and with fewer interruptions. Research shows that people who exercise tend to have better sleep patterns. Better sleep can lead to a wide number of benefits on health and wellbeing, including decreased headaches and sugar cravings, better moods, less pain, and overall feeling better.

The endorphins released by exercise also lower the risk and symptoms of depression. Strength training may not cure depression, but it can improve your quality of life. Even if you don't have depression, strength training can help prevent you from becoming depressed. These endorphins make you, generally, a happier person overall.

As we age, our thinking processes and brain activity slow. This increases the risk of dementia and Alzheimer's. Strength training keeps the mind and body active. A consistently active mind can have reduced risks of Alzheimer's and dementia.

It's no secret that our joints become stiff and painful. The fluid that helps our joints slide past each other decreases as we get older. Think of a door hinge that needs to be oiled. Exercise can improve the fluid in our joints, making them less stiff and easier to move. Exercise also strengthens muscles and tendons surrounding joints, improving pain. This shows why exercise can increase quality of life through improving function and mobility. This can help keep you from becoming depressed and socially isolated.

SIGNS AND SYMPTOMS

Chronic conditions cause pain and problems in our everyday lives. The signs and symptoms from illnesses can create as many problems as the illness itself. Strength training can improve signs and symptoms associated with several conditions. Some common problems that can be improved through exercise are (Seguin et al., 2002; Rizzo, 2021):

- Arthritis. Osteoarthritis can lead to less flexibility, pain, and stiffness. Strength training reduces stiffness and pain while increasing flexibility and strength. Improved function and reduction in disability are some benefits you can expect.
- Diabetes. Diabetes is the body's inability to control blood sugar and/or insulin secretion. Strength training is shown to improve glycemic control, reduce fasting blood sugar levels, reduce HbA1c, and decrease the dosage of required medications.
- Osteoporosis. Obesity, poor bone density, previous injuries, muscle weakness, and joint problems can lead to osteoporosis. When you strength train bones and muscles strengthen leading to less risk of fractures and injury after falls.
- Back pain. Strength training strengthens stomach and back muscles, which can reduce stress on the spine and improve pain and movement.

- Heart disease. Exercise is shown to improve lipid profiles and overall fitness, which contributes to heart health. Improved muscle mass is also a benefit and can improve the risk of death in patients with heart disease.
- Obesity. Obesity is a risk factor as we age. Our metabolism slows, leading to fewer calories being burned and more storage of fat. Strength training can help maintain weight loss, lose weight, improve metabolism, and burn calories.
- Cardiovascular function. As we age, the cells that control heart pace and rigidity of the heart deteriorate. This has a negative effect on blood flow and circulation. Strength training can prevent and slow the deterioration of these cells.
- Lower lung capacity and strength. Lung capacity and strength is the lung's ability to hold, intake, and use oxygen. Exercise training can strengthen the lungs and improve the management and flow of oxygen.
- Increased blood pressure. Due to the benefits to the heart, strength training can decrease systolic and diastolic blood pressure (or the top and bottom numbers on a blood pressure reading).
- Decreased muscle endurance and strength. Muscle endurance is the ability to continuously work for a period of time. Strength is the ability to move the

body and lift weight. Strength training improves muscle endurance and strength.

- Inflammation. Inflammation is the swelling of tissues in the body. Exercise improves blood and water flow in the body, improving inflammation.
- Inflexibility. Inflexibility can lead to falls, pain, stiffness, and more. Increased joint fluid and blood flow improves flexibility in older adults. Strength training also lets muscles release tension that can cause inflexibility.
- Brain dysfunctions. Cognitive (brain) function slows as we age. However, this can be decreased and stopped through strength training. The improvement in mood, stress, sleep, blood flow and oxygen contribute to positive changes in brain dysfunctions caused by old age.

MOTIVATION

Motivation plays a large role in strength training. Both internal and external motivations can help you stick with your training. Morio Higaonna acts as a role model for Japanese citizens. Morio is an 83-year-old karate instructor. Yes, you read that correctly. Born in 1938, Morio still practices and teaches karate today. From a young age, Morio understood the benefits and importance of exercise, physical activity, and strength training. Morio can be your motivation to get started. If he can, you can!

Journaling your exercises can also motivate you to keep going. Journaling your exercise means writing down the exercise you did, how many times you did it, whether or not you used weight, and how much weight was used. Journaling exercises have been shown to help you learn your workout faster, remember your progress, and keep track of where you started. You can buy a Workout Journal or use a smart-phone app to collect and write down your exercises. Journaling will also act as motivation to keep you exercising.

If you believe that strength training can yield the desired changes that you want to see in your life then you must start working out. Are you confused about where to start? Don't worry chapter by chapter we have got you covered. The next chapter helps you get started!

2

ROLL THE BALL AND KEEP IT ROLLING

Making the choice to get active is one of the most beneficial activities you can do to improve your health and happiness. As with anything in our lives, deciding to start or making a change can be scary and overwhelming. Don't worry! We're going to cover some common worries about exercising, how to properly get started, what to wear, and how to handle muscle soreness after training. Think of where you'll be just a few weeks from now!

Motivation is the match that starts the fire. However, you need wood to keep it going. Motivation is enough to get started, but effectively working out means staying disciplined. You have to make the choice to work on yourself and be better than you were yesterday.

Strength training can sound scary if you haven't had much experience, so it's important we talk about some of the common worries surrounding exercise and physical activity.

"I'm going to fall or get hurt."

Fear of falling is a big concern that will hold people back. However, many exercise programs can help prevent falls from happening. You will learn relevant, beneficial exercises that strengthen the muscles that help you keep and regain your balance. Falls often happen because muscles across the body are weakened, meaning they cannot contract and help you catch yourself. They may also react too slowly, meaning you're already falling before you can catch yourself. Strength training will help your muscles move stronger and faster, keeping you from going down.

"It's going to be too hard."

Exercise doesn't have to be painful. Some can associate strength training with big muscle gains or hurting yourself. While strength training is meant to work your muscles, over time the exercises will become easier as you become stronger. It doesn't always have to be "no pain, no gain". You can still build and tone your muscles through light strength training.

"I have health problems."

Oftentimes, seniors report being hesitant to exercise because of tiredness, lack of willpower, poor health, and pain. Some worry about heart attack and stroke during exercise. Dealing with conditions can be tough when trying to exercise and hold some back. Fear of making these problems worse can prevent you from reaching your best self.

Getting strong social support can help you when you need it. It can be especially difficult to work out if you've had a rough day, if you're tired, or if you're dealing with problems from other conditions. Having a social support network will help you overcome the sadness and loss of motivation that comes with symptoms and health issues. Social support networks can be friends, family, neighbors, coworkers, and other influential people that you see regularly.

"I don't know where to start."

Getting started can be one of the hardest parts. Lack of confidence means not being confident in your abilities to lift weights and make the changes for a healthier lifestyle. Seniors can have poor self-confidence, which can keep them from testing their limits and taking on a new program. Learning how to start exercising will set you up for success.

"I don't have time."

Sometimes a difference in personal and professional agendas can hold people back. Sometimes having responsibilities from your family, such as babysitting a grandchild, can act as a barrier to exercise. Working out can give you more energy, meaning you can make the most out of your time. Exercise can improve productivity, which can open up some time for you to train.

"I won't fit in. It'll be awkward."

It has been shown that older adults tend to feel self-conscious and awkward when working out, especially in front of younger and stronger people. Having no experience with exercise also leads to low self-esteem. Having to watch someone else teach you how to perform the exercises can be awkward for some. Exercising with peers can help you overcome this feeling of social awkwardness. Interacting with others will also increase your social support and keep you from feeling depressed, isolated, and lonely. Exercising at home can be comfortable, private, and boost confidence. If working out in a group or with others is a goal for you, you can do it! Exercise at home until you feel confident enough to meet up with others.

Doctor's Orders

Although strength training is beneficial, if you're over 50 and/or have little experience exercising, you must talk to your doctor before starting a routine. This is to help you stay safe and effective.

One workout or activity doesn't fit all. Different workouts are beneficial for different people. They will be able to help you determine what exercises you can do, and which ones will be the most beneficial for you. Meeting with a physician also allows them to find any underlying conditions or problems that could keep you from working out. This way, you can perform the workouts that you're able to do safely. Your doctor will also help you look at your personality and responsibilities to find the workouts that best fit your current lifestyle. You don't have to change everything just to add strength training into your life!

What would you like to accomplish from working out? What is one thing in your life that you'd like to be able to do easier? Meeting with your doctor will help you determine your goals and needs as a senior. Having goals is going to help you get started. Setting goals allows you to find a plan that will be easiest to incorporate into your lifestyle.

Typically, a physician performs a physical before suggesting any type of exercise or strength training programs. This physical allows you to see a great starting point. Your physician could also order a blood test to rule out any potential harm or conditions. You can use this as motivation and a guide when sticking with your routine. The results from before and after exercising will be evident from these tests. You will be able to find any potential risks and obstacles, as well. Before exercising, you should tell your physician if you have any of the following:

- Discomfort or pain in the neck, jaw, arms, and/or chests during physical activity
- Fainting or dizziness
- Shortness of breath with little movement, such as when going to bed.
- Swelling of the ankles, especially at nighttime
- Rapid or strong heartbeat
- Lower leg pain that disappears with rest
- Heart murmur or other problems

You should see a physician before beginning an exercise program if 2 or more of the following apply to you (Cheung et al., 2003):

You have not exercised for a minimum of 30 minutes, at least 3 days a week, for three or more months.

- Men with a family history of heart disease before 55, and 65 in women.
- If you're older than 45 for a man and 55 for a woman.
- You are a current smoker, or you've stopped within the past 6 months.
- High cholesterol and blood pressure.
- Obesity or overweight.
- Prediabetes.

WHAT SHOULD I ASK?

Meeting with a doctor about exercise can be overwhelming with all the information being given to you at once. While at your appointment, be sure to ask some important questions to get the information you need.

- Do I need to avoid any certain activities or exercise?

What works for someone else could be harmful to you, and vice versa. Your doctor will use your health history, current conditions, and physical or blood work to make recommendations. This is also a good opportunity for you to tell the doctor about any new or worsening symptoms.

- Do I need any preventative care?

It's important to partake in preventative care as we age to keep ourselves healthy and independent. Preventative care, including women over 65 being checked for osteoporosis, should be assessed, and completed before starting an exercise program.

- Does my condition affect my exercise?

Conditions and symptoms can be irritated by exercise. For example, during times of a flare-up, patients with arthritis should avoid certain exercises to avoid making them worse. Seniors with diabetes may need to change their eating and/or insulin schedule to accommodate exercise. Finding out how your conditions affect your workout sets you up to start exercising more safely.

WHAT SHOULD I WEAR?

Proper clothes and footwear are important for ensuring they don't affect your workout. This would include wearing a dress or long pants, or flip flops or slippers. The dress or pants could cause you to trip and the sandals and slippers could leave your feet prone to injuries from dropping weights or other equipment you may be using. They also don't allow for much support for your feet, making it harder to get a better workout.

There's no reason why older adults need to dress any differently than other ages when working out. Shorts, skorts, leggings, and joggers are all acceptable for exercising. Older women tend to want to cover more, so a tunic or long shirt over leggings can be comfortable and effective to train in. Hoodies, jackets, and vests can be worn when it's colder and tank tops and t-shirts can be worn when it's warmer. If you tend to stay cold, you can warm up in a hoodie or sweater. Once you get warm you can take it off.

Silk undergarments and clothing shouldn't be worn, as well as clothes that don't fit properly. Silk can cause you to get too hot or slide off a chair you may be using. Clothing with extra material, such as robes and ruffles, shouldn't be worn, as it can get stuck in equipment.

Finding a fabric you like to wear during your workout depends on what the workout is and what you're looking for in your clothes. For example, some clothing can pull the sweat from your body, allowing it to dry faster. When you are going to sweat a lot, finding wicking fabric, such as polypropylene, can be good for keeping you dry and comfortable. Cotton, however, absorbs sweat, making it feel wet and heavy. Rubber or plastic-based materials can make your body sweat more and stay hot longer. Overall, your clothing shouldn't interfere with your movement or workout.

INDOOR VERSUS OUTDOOR

Training outdoors requires certain clothing and fabric for you to get the best workout. When working out in the outdoors, make sure your outfits are changing with the seasons. During warmer weather, it's important to use a material that allows airflow and pulls away sweat. These clothes should be cool and comfortable and let you move easier.

When you're exercising, you naturally raise your body temperature. This can be beneficial when training in the colder months but may be too warm if you've dressed for cold weather. Dressing in layers is beneficial because if you start to get too warm you can take something off. You can wear a long sleeve with a zip-up jacket or vest. Always dress warmer than you think you will need and ensure your hands, ears, and head are covered in colder temperatures. Wearing layers can also help protect you from wind and rain.

FOOTWEAR

Footwear is an important part of strength and balance training. Footwear can help maintain balance, prevent injury, and correct form so you're doing the exercise properly. It can be overwhelming to try and find the right footwear. There are so many brands, sizes, shapes, and colors to choose from. You can meet with a podiatrist or physical therapist to help you determine which shoe will be best. You can choose your shoes based on:

- The type of exercise. Different exercises require different types of shoes. Dancing, walking, or running can put strain on your joints. Having more support for these types of exercises is important for preventing pain.
- Amount of support. Daily walks wouldn't require as much foot and ankle support as running. A minimalist shoe will be flimsy and have little interior padding.

More support means having a firmer outer shell and enough padding to absorb the impact from your foot hitting the ground. If you're unsure, getting a shoe with more support is a safe way to go.

- Wear current shoes. If you look at the bottom of shoes you commonly wear, you will see wear marks either on the front, back, or outer sides of the shoe. This shows you the areas on your feet where you put the most pressure. For example, if you have more wear on the heels of your feet, you'll want to make sure the soles of your new shoes are thick in the heel.

- Arch support and foot shape. Every foot shape is different. Some people have high arches and others may have a flat foot. Knowing your foot shape and arch size can help you choose the shoes that are best for you. Visiting a running shoe store can also help you find the best shoes.

- Style and comfort. Buying shoes that look good will make you feel good. Stylish shoes will motivate you to want to put them on and train. Your shoes should be comfortable, as well.

What you wear, on your body and feet, can decide whether or not you have a safe and enjoyable workout. Once you've chosen your attire, you can gather any equipment you have or need for a great training session.

EQUIPMENT

You don't have to have expensive or fancy equipment to get an effective workout. Some of the best workouts have come from reusing a plastic bottle. Filling two-liter bottles, or empty gallon jugs, with sand or water can create anywhere from 4 – 12 pounds. Rinse out any plastic bottles with lids that you have. Fill them with water or sand using a funnel and duct tape or glue the lid shut.

A kettlebell is a weighted sphere with a handle. You can recreate kettlebells by using bags and food items. Take a bag and fill it with heavy items, such as canned foods or bags of rice, and fill it up with enough weight that you want. Tie the bag in a tight knot and place it inside a second bag. Tie the second bag tightly but leave enough room on the handles for you to grasp. Now you have a weighted bag that you can use the same way as a kettlebell. Paint cans and bags of onions or apples can also be used as a kettlebell.

Ankle weights can be attached to the ankles and used to add resistance to different exercises. You can make your own ankle weights with sand or rice, socks, and shoelaces. Fill each sock with rice or sand. Leave some fabric on either side of the rice or sand and tie it closed with a shoelace. Wrap the sock around your ankle, then tie the shoelace around and into a bow. This works best with long socks.

Dumbbells are short weights with an area for you to grab to lift. There are many items that can be used in place of dumbbells. Laundry detergent, canned or jarred foods, and even water bottles can be used to work your arms. Smaller items should fit in your hand (water bottle) and larger ones should have a handle for you to grasp (laundry detergent). Make sure, if you've made your weights, that they are all sealed. When measuring out and using dumbbells, try to make sure they're equal in weight. You want to get the same workout on both arms. If one is heavier than the other, that arm will get more of a workout than the other.

Sandbags are exactly what they sound like: bags of sand. As you can imagine, you can make your own. Find a liner bag that you can use to seal in the sand, such as a trash bag or zipper freezer bag. Leave room for the sand to move around or else it could put too much pressure on the liner and cause rips and tears. Then place that bag inside another. You can now use it for squats, bicep curls, and more. You can also use wood pellets, rubber mulch, and pea gravel in place of sand.

A barbell is a long bar with weights on either end. You can recreate barbells at home by using metal rods or bars with gallon containers on the end. You can use a broomstick with the broom end detached, for example. You can fill these containers with gravel, water, or sand, attach them to each end with duct tape or zip ties, and use the pole to lift and control them.

There are a number of items around the house that can be used to exercise, without needing to alter them. Using books can be a great way to add some weight to a workout without having to create anything. You can use books to curl up to train your arms or hold for squats.

You can create and collect exercise equipment in several creative ways. You can repurpose bottles or grab heavier items around the house to use to give your muscles a better workout. A better workout could motivate you to keep going.

STAYING MOTIVATED

It's common to lose the motivation to exercise. Tiredness, medical conditions, and a busy schedule can diminish the motivation to train. Sometimes exercise will be the last thing on your mind. However, there are many simple things you can remember to make your workouts more enjoyable and manageable.

- *Make it fun.* Doing the same exercise routine can get boring and lead to burnout. When you find activities you like, you're going to want to keep training. You can simply do what you normally do, just add weight or do it quicker. Making exercise more enjoyable can be done in many ways.

o Walk on the golf course instead of taking the cart.

o Park towards the back of the parking lot of your favorite store, so you have a longer walk to the store and back to your car.

o Sign up for a dance class. You could even bring a partner.

o Walk a nature trail and stop for photos or to identify plants and birds. Keep a journal of what you see.

o Walk around the mall.

o Schedule a training or exercise date with a friend.

o Go swimming or ride your bike through the neighborhood.

- *Socialize.* People are more likely to stick with their program when they have people working with them. Having good people around you can also motivate you to get the job done. Even if you're homebound, you can use the computer to set up virtual meetings and posts to gather people to cheer you on. Telling others about your goals also keeps you accountable. You can walk with coworkers for lunch or play outdoor activities at a family function.

- *Think of the benefits.* We've discussed some of the physical and mental benefits of exercise. Imagine a day when your pain is almost gone. Think of having enough energy to get through a busy day. Consider how much better you will feel. Visualize the stronger, healthier you and work towards getting there.

- *Set goals.* It can be overwhelming when moving from no exercise to 30 minutes a day. Setting small, attainable goals can keep you motivated to keep going. Start with a 10-minute walk after lunch. After a few weeks, turn it into a 15-minute walk. Then 20 minutes. After some time, you will be walking 30-minutes a day. Setting these milestones, instead of jumping straight to 30 minutes, can be encouraging while training.

- *Track your progress.* Use a journal or app to keep track of your progress. Focusing on how far you've come can be great for your mindset. Wearable fitness trackers can increase activity levels. Tracking your progress can be fun when you give yourself small rewards after reaching a milestone. For example, check your progress journal every week. If you do strength training for fifteen minutes a day, three times a week, treat yourself to a hot bath or a new book. Tracking your progress also shows you where you're able to get the most exercise.

- *Fit exercise into your daily activities.* Do you normally walk the dog, babysit your grandchildren, or go grocery shopping? Try walking the dog longer or slightly faster than normal. You can play a game outdoors with your grandchildren or aim to walk down every aisle at the store. You can incorporate exercises however it works for you and reward yourself when you do them. Take yourself to a movie, go out to eat, or get a massage.

Staying motivated takes patience and self-discipline. It also means persevering through obstacles to get physically active. It is common to be sore after exercise. Sometimes this can make you want to skip your planned activity. It's important to understand the difference between pain and delayed onset muscle soreness.

DELAYED ONSET MUSCLE SORENESS

When we exercise, we are working muscles past the point of their normal workload. This creates microscopic tears in the muscle tissue. This is what causes your muscles to be sore (Sarnataro & DerSarkissian, 2022). When they grow back to normal, they'll be stronger than before.

Even the best athletes can experience DOMS. Delayed-onset muscle soreness, or DOMS, is muscle pain that starts after exercise. You won't experience DOMS during your workout, but you can expect to feel it 1 – 2 days after exercise. The burning sensation that you feel during exercise is caused by working the muscles. This typically stops soon after exercising.

DOMS can make it hard to stay on track with your program. DOMS can feel the worst from 1 – 3 days after training but typically goes down with time. You may be experiencing DOMS if you have:

- Tender muscles
- Stiffness and pain when moving, leading to reducing mobility.
- Swelling
- Muscle fatigue
- Short-term strength loss

DOMS is most noticeable when you start exercising after being inactive for a long time. How long and hard you work out will also determine DOMS. You can use nonsteroidal anti-inflammatory drugs (NSAIDs) to help with soreness. Heat has also been shown to be beneficial. Exercise can actually be the best remedy for DOMS, although the effects may be short-lived. Reducing the intensity of your workout in the 1 – 2 days after tough exercise can help with DOMS.

Areas of the body that aren't as sore should be worked on after DOMS. For example, if your arms are pretty sore after a work-out, you can spend that day working on your legs. Introducing exercise to your life over a 1 – 2-week timeframe can help prevent DOMS from being too painful.

Having a cool-down phase after your program helps DOMS from being too severe. Usually this can include a light stretch, a short walk, and deep breaths. After you deal with DOMS, the next time you perform those exercises it'll be easier for you because you'll be stronger.

Because you get stronger each time you do the set of exercises that caused DOMS, it's important to cross-train so you work different muscles. You can do this by switching up the muscle groups that you're working on. You can work the lower legs instead of the upper legs.

Rest days can be very important to improving DOMS. Taking adequate rest days can prevent your DOMS from causing pain, not discomfort. Rest days are the time for you to rest your muscles so they can recuperate. Rest when you can, take a warm bath or shower, and avoid any intense movement or exercise.

If you notice that your DOMS is painful or it's interfering with your daily activities, it may be time to slow down. Decrease the time or intensity of your workout until your DOMS is uncomfortable, not painful. If the pain doesn't go away, set up an appointment with your doctor.

Meeting with your doctor before beginning exercise is beneficial for preventing injury and improving motivation. Your doctor will be able to tell you what exercises you can do safely. They will also advise on the best exercises for you and help you set goals. Your doctor can also help you with some basic strength training advice when needed. In the next chapter we are going to learn about the basics of strength training. We are now quickly approaching our training sessions.

3

ESSENTIALS OF STRENGTH TRAINING

Knowing the basics of strength training allows you to understand how to perform an exercise program safely, prevent injury, and better reach your goals. The main part of understanding strength training means understanding how to work the correct muscles in the correct way, and when to rest them.

Rest is just as important as training. Understanding when to rest helps keep your muscles healthy. Understanding the importance of rest means knowing about the basic principles of strength training: overload, progression and specificity.

OVERLOAD

Your friend Miller started an exercise program a few weeks ago. He was telling you how much he enjoyed it and how he could already tell a difference in his strength. After a while though, he started to complain that his success had plateaued, and he noticed he wasn't getting any stronger than the week before. He didn't know what he was doing wrong.

Overload means putting more stress on a muscle than what it's used to. After Miller had been doing those exercises consistently for a while, his muscles became accustomed to those movements. His muscles were no longer being overloaded.

For his training to be successful, he needs to increase the intensity or duration of his workouts. His muscles are going to be overloaded again, leading to an increase in strength. If he has been doing 10 squats, 10 bicep curls, and a 10-minute walk, he would need to do more squats and bicep curls and/or increase the length of his walk. It's important not to move up too fast, as it could cause DOMS or injury.

PROGRESSION

After his muscles become accustomed to his new routine, they will stop being overloaded. This means he will continuously have to gradually improve his workout. This is called progression. Moving up in weights or reps every so often can ensure the muscles are still being overloaded, leading to strength increases. When focusing on progression and overload, Miller should remember FITT.

- Frequency – number of times training each week.
- Intensity – how hard you work out.
- Time – how long your training lasts.
- Type – the kind of training.

Altering a workout can be done in several ways. For Miller to keep getting his strength gains, he needs to alter his workout through the above principles. He can increase the number of times he works out, make it harder, longer, or do different types of training. You can alter your workout and make it harder or easier by changing these aspects.

SPECIFICITY

Specificity is the idea that adaptations occur as a result of stress placed on sections of the body and only on these sections. Specificity refers to the muscle groups trained, training speed, training intensity, movements, and energy systems used. Gaining strength and speed can be done by working the same muscle groups in different ways.

If Miller wanted to be able to walk faster, he could perform exercises that work similar muscle groups that walking requires. He could do lunges, squats, or leg curls. He could also do leg lifts and calf raises. Strength training the same muscle groups required for a certain activity can improve effectiveness and productivity.

TYPES OF RESISTANCE TRAINING

Resistance is the use of an object or movement that requires the muscle to flex or contract. Resistance training can lead to increases in strength and power. Different forms of resistance training include:

- *Free weights.* This is the use of dumbbells, kettlebells, or other household items created with weight. Think back to the jugs of sand and the full water bottles for dumbbells.
- *Sandbags or medicine balls.* These can be used to perform exercises by adding weight to increase resistance. Increasing resistance leads to increased strength gains.
- *Weight machines.* Exercise equipment is beneficial for guiding exercises and ensuring safety when used correctly. Handles and adjustable seats make the machines more comfortable and safer.
- *Resistance bands.* Think of large, wide rubber bands that you can place around your arms or legs. Moving against these tight bands makes your muscles work hard enough to be overloaded.
- *Suspension equipment.* This equipment is a tool that uses body weight and gravity to perform many resistance exercises.

- *Body weight.* Your body weight can be a great part of resistance training. Push-ups, chin-ups, and squats can be very beneficial to training and you don't need any equipment.

While there is a wide array of benefits that come from resistance training, working the same muscle groups every day can be harmful, painful, and could lead to injuries. Lifting weights every day can be done, but you must ensure you're not working the same muscle groups day after day.

Your muscles need time to rebuild and repair between bouts of exercise. Without rest, they cannot repair appropriately. You can alternate muscle groups each day, so you don't hurt yourself. You can work your arms one day, then your legs the next. Taking 2 – 3 days between muscle groups can allow your muscles to repair more effectively.

SEVEN MAJOR MUSCLE GROUPS

There are seven major groups of muscles that you should alternate when exercising: chest, back, shoulders, biceps, triceps, core, and lower body. When there is not enough time for rest, these muscle groups cannot be repaired together. It's best to only target a few muscle groups at a time. Many people find it easier to work muscle groups that are closer together each time. So, someone would exercise their shoulders, chest, and biceps one day, and focus on their core and lower body the next.

Grouping muscle groups together can be a way to mix up your workouts. If you're exercising three times a week, you could work chest and shoulders on day one, legs on day two, and back, arms, and abdominals on day three. If you're lifting twice a week, you can do arms, chest, and shoulders on day one, then legs, back, and abdominals on day two. Focusing on these main muscle groups will help you improve your program and your fitness. If Miller wanted to squat with more weight, he would want to do legs and back on one day, then core on another.

Training certain muscle groups together can increase effectiveness and fitness level. Think of the bicep in a bicep curl. You're focusing on contracting your bicep. However, the muscles in your shoulders are also being used. Cycling between muscle groups for your training days can allow for adequate rest and repair. It can be more beneficial to think about working that one muscle group because you will get to rest that group in the days to come.

EXERCISES FOR EACH GROUP

There are several exercises that can be completed to target each muscle group. The exercises may sound unfamiliar or intimidating, but you'll learn about each exercise and how to perform it correctly with descriptions and pictures.

1. Chest

- Bench press
- Incline and decline bench press
- Dumbbell bench press
- Dumbbell fly
- Chest dip
- Seated machine press
- Incline dumbbell bench press

2. Arms (Biceps and Triceps)

- Tricep pushdowns and extensions
- Close grip bench press
- Dumbbell, barbell, and hammer curls
- Pushups

3. Back

- Bent rows
- Barbell and dumbbell rows
- Deadlift
- Pullups and chin-ups
- Cable or machine rows
- Kettlebell swings

- Front squats
- Lat pull-downs

4. Abs/Core

- Sit-ups
- Crunches
- Bicycle crunches
- Mountain climbers
- Scissor raises
- Plank and side plank
- Lateral crawls
- Seated twists
- Leg raises

5. Legs

- Lunges
- Squats
- Stair steppers
- Deadlift
- Box jumps
- Sumo squats
- Hip bridges
- Toe raises
- Leg press

6. Shoulders

- Lateral press
- Seated shoulder press
- Overhead shoulder press
- Bent over dumbbell lateral raises
- Standing shrugs

REPETITIONS, SETS, AND REST INTERVALS

Depending on your goals, your workout program will differ in weight, repetitions, sets, rest intervals, and speed. Repetitions, or reps, are one full contraction and relaxation of the muscle. This would be one crunch, one bicep curl, one pushup, or one lunge. A max rep is the most you can lift or move in one repetition.

For example, a water bottle would be comfortable for you (2 pounds), and a full laundry detergent bottle could be the most you can lift (5 pounds). When choosing weight, it's important that you keep the correct form. If you notice your form is starting to waiver, lower the amount of weight. If the max number of reps you could do in one set is 12, your rep max would be 12.

A set is several repetitions grouped together. A set could be 8 crunches, 10 pushups, or 12 arm raises. In a workout program, you typically do one exercise for 3 – 5 sets. You could tell

Miller in order to get stronger, he could do 10 reps of squats for 3 sets, with rest in between each set.

Rest is just as important as the number of reps and sets in an exercise program. Rest between sets is important for letting your muscles return to normal before starting again. Between sets, it's important to rest from 30 seconds to 2 minutes. If you've recently increased intensity or duration, longer rest periods between sets may be more beneficial for you. Some exercises may need longer rest times than others. Your goals can also determine the amount of rest.

- If your goal is strength, lift heavier weights for fewer reps, with 2 – 5 minutes of rest between sets.
- If you want to make your muscles larger or more defined, spend 30 – 60 seconds of rest.
- Muscle endurance, or the ability to do more reps, should have a rest time of 30 – 60 seconds between sets.

RECOVERY AND REST DAY WORKOUTS

While exercise is shown to prevent injuries, exercising inappropriately can lead to injury. Do enough reps and sets to challenge your muscles, but not so much that it starts to hurt or put a strain on the wrong areas. It is recommended that your progress should be made from no exercise to three times a week, across a 6-month time span.

Here is a list of training recommendations, precautions, and goals:

- Start your training slowly and work up.
- Don't train the same muscle groups two days in a row.
- Increase weight and resistance over time.
- Performs reps with controlled, slow movements.
- Stretch your arms and legs out and use the full range of motion in each joint.
- When exerting, or pushing, breathe out. Don't ever hold your breath.
- If you experience shortness of breath, chest discomfort, joint pain, dizziness, or heart palpitations then you should stop the exercise.

Rest and recovery are important parts of exercising, especially for older adults who are strength training. Knowing about rest, and the best exercises for you can help you be a more effective trainer. Let's discuss some of the best exercises seniors can perform.

4

STRETCHING YOUR TOES

There's not one exercise that will work alone to reach all of your goals. Mixing activities throughout the week can help you get the most from your workout routine. Creating a balanced exercise plan is as beneficial as a balanced diet. A balanced exercise plan consists of:

- 150 minutes of moderate-intensity activity (3o minutes a day, five times a week)
- 2 – 3 strength training sessions a week with at least 48 hours of rest between sessions for muscle recovery.
- Balance exercises to prevent falls (Cavill & Foster, 2018).

This can sound daunting, but you can break your workout up into multiple times a day. You can strength train for 30 minutes or take two 15-minute walks. Each time you work out you should have a warm-up and a cool-down. When cooling down, simply slow down your activity or lower intensity a few minutes before stopping and stretching afterward. A balanced exercise plan is a healthy mixture of different types of exercises. Whether you're in the gym, at home, using weights, or only body weight, some exercises are especially beneficial for older adults.

Aerobic exercise, or cardio, is great for losing fat and burning calories. Cardio consists of biking, running, walking, and swimming. Aerobic exercise boosts short-term breathing and heart rate. This allows more oxygen to reach the muscles and improves cardiovascular endurance. This type of exercise is associated with lowering the risk of diseases and having a longer life span.

Strength training is a beneficial part of an exercise program. Strength training can protect against bone loss and build muscle. It can tone your muscles, improve your muscle-to-fat ratio, and make daily activities easier. It's recommended that you should perform strength training at least twice a week with a 48-hour rest period between working a certain muscle group. One set per exercise session will suffice, but 2 – 3 sets per exercise can be more effective. Here are a few tips when strength training:

- **Pay attention to your form, not the weight.** Your body should be aligned correctly and move through the motions smoothly. Poor form can lead to a strain on tendons and other tissues. When starting with a new type of exercise, begin with no weight so your body can get accustomed to the movements before adding weight.
- **Keep pace.** Keeping the same tempo throughout the rep can ensure you're working the right muscles. As an example, if you're doing a bench press then count to 5 while lifting a dumbbell, hold for 2 seconds, then count to 5 as you lower it down.
- **Breathe while doing your exercises.** Holding your breath could lead to dizziness or fainting. Exhale as you push, pull, or lift and inhale as you release. If you're having trouble not holding your breath, count your tempo out loud. You can't hold your breath if you're speaking.
- **Keep challenging your muscles.** You'll want to pick a weight that causes you to tire out on the last two sets while keeping your form. If you're unable to do the normal number of reps, switch to a lower weight.

Balance exercises can be especially helpful for older adults. It is normal for balance to get worse as we age, but that doesn't mean we have to let it go completely downhill. Many medications and conditions may cause dizziness, numbness, tingling, and pain which can all decrease balance. Poor balance can lead to falls and injuries. However, there are exercises you can add to your program to improve your balance.

- **Walking.** Walking can strengthen the muscles in the legs and ankles that are responsible for holding your foot and ankle in place while walking. Strengthening these muscles can help you keep your balance by keeping you steadier.
- **Pilates.** Pilates is a low-intensity workout that strengthens muscles, improves posture, and enhances flexibility.
- **Core exercises.** Our balance is affected by our core. Our core is the muscles around our stomach and sides that are used for all movements and exercises. If we have weak cores, it's going to be easier for us to fall. Working muscles in the back will also assist the core in keeping our balance.

Balance exercises should be done within the recommended 30 minutes a day or muscle strengthening and balance training, three times a week. You can also include at least 30 minutes of walking twice or more each week. Improving balance is going to help improve flexibility.

Flexibility can be enhanced through stretching. Flexibility is the body's ability to move in a full range of motion across all joints. Muscles get shorter and tighter as we age, so it's important to focus on flexibility as a senior. Short, stiff muscles can lead to pain, balance problems, and injuries.

Frequently stretching muscles and surrounding tissues fight the negative effects of aging on the muscles. When muscles are adequately stretched, it is easier to achieve a full range of motion. This will improve performance and functional abilities. Stretching is also beneficial for improving mood and blood flow. Stretching can be a great way to start the day or wind down in the evening.

Stretching as a cool-down is a great way to improve flexibility. The frequency of flexibility exercises is up to each person. It is suggested that older adults should complete flexibility exercises with strength activities or aerobic exercise, at least twice a week. Strengthening our core can improve strength training, balance, and flexibility.

FORM

Tevin and Marcus go into the gym and decide to set a friendly competition. Whoever had improved the most in arm strength by the end of the month would have to buy dinner. Tevin started at 5-pound bicep curls, 8 reps, for 2 sets. Marcus did the same. The next week, Tevin decided to move to 8-pounds, 8 reps, for 2 sets. Marcus stayed with 5-pounds but moved up to 10 reps. The next week Tevin moved to 10 pounds and Marcus moved to 8. At the end of the month, both were asked to complete as many reps as they could with a 5-pound weight. After a few reps, Tevin starts to complain of elbow pain and decides to stop, leaving Marcus victorious.

Having the correct form means completing the exercise in the correct motions while using the appropriate muscles. Having improper form could lead to injury or decreased effectiveness. Because Tevin moved up too fast in weight, his form faltered in order to compensate for the energy needed for the increase in weight. Although he was using 10-pound weights, Marcus was able to perform the reps longer because his form was strong. If the weight is too much, it can cause muscles and tendons to stress themselves to lift the weight. This puts pressure on the wrong parts of the body.

To improve your form, you can:

Talk with a trainer. Even if you cannot hire a personal trainer, many gyms and programs offer employees who can help answer your questions. Having someone watch you perform exercises also provides an outside view. This is something you can't get by watching yourself. They will be able to give advice and make recommendations on how to improve your form.

- **Warm-up.** Warming up before you start allows your muscles to loosen and receive more blood flow before using them to exercise. Warming up will decrease the chance of injury.

- **Start with little to no weight.** Getting accustomed to the movement before adding weight can ensure you're using the right form. Plus, you will feel how the exercise is supposed to feel. That way, when you're exercising you will know if you're doing it with the correct form or not, depending on your feeling.
- **Visualize the exercise.** There is a mind-muscle connection. Think about the muscle groups that you're working on. Focus on how the muscles feel. If the muscle you're supposed to be working on doesn't feel like it should, you could have improper form.
- **Use muscles, not momentum.** It can be easy to just swing your arm up and down from momentum. However, this can lead to flimsy movements and less effectiveness. Use your muscles to contract and release, moving the body smoothly and pausing occasionally (such as at the top of a bicep curl).
- **Stand up straight.** Slouching can have a negative effect on your form. Slouching can make certain muscles short and tight and decrease blood flow in certain areas. Hold your stomach in and roll your shoulders back. Hunching your shoulders can lead to tight muscles in the neck. Imagine someone is holding you up with a string on the top of your head. Lengthening the spine helps your posture.

- **Breathe.** Holding your breath can cause the muscles in your chest and back to tighten. Inhale through the nose and exhale through the mouth to relax your shoulders. Let them drop and focus on your breath going into your stomach.
- **Listen to your body.** Even if you're using the same weight, if you're experiencing DOMS or a flare-up of a condition, it's okay to lower weight or reps. Working through soreness is different than working through pain.

Focusing on proper form maximizes workout efficiency and minimizes the risk of injury. Your form can be improved through warming up and stretching.

WARMING UP

Amber woke up and decided to do some strength exercises before starting her day. She rolled out of bed, laid on the ground, and began doing her exercises. After ten minutes, she stands up and heads out to start her day. About an hour later, she starts to feel sore, and her joints are hurting more than normal.

Amber should have started with a small warm-up, even if she was only going to do 10 minutes of exercise. She could have walked or jogged in place for two minutes, performed leg lifts, or body weight bicep curls. Afterward, she could have done some toe touches and arm stretches to help her body cool down from exercise. Had this been done, she could have avoided the soreness and joint pain.

Warming up is beneficial for many reasons. However, if you warm up or stretch incorrectly, it could lead to injury or decreased effectiveness. Warming up allows you to improve your range of motion and avoid injury. Warming up the muscles allows their fibers to become more elastic, similar to a rubber band. This allows you to get a better workout.

You should perform a full body warm-up, even if you're only working on certain muscle groups. If you're working on a certain body part, you can do more warmups associated with that area. However, be sure to include some other muscles, as they are all connected, and it can help overall performance.

As you get closer to your workout your warmup should increase in intensity. This also allows your heart to warm up to the exercise. Your warmup should consist of gentle exercises that lead to active stretches that combine movements and stretching. After stretching you can begin to increase in weight and intensity.

STRETCHING

When stretching, it's important to warm up first. Stretching muscles that aren't warmed up can lead to strain and injury. After warming up, it's time to move towards stretching. Slow, controlled dynamic stretching is like "bouncing" while sitting down and reaching for your toes. It includes arm circles and hip rotations and other activities such as Pilates. Some stretches that are beneficial for the lower body are knee lifts, butt kicks, and taking long-stride steps.

Static stretches, or going into a stretch and holding it, should be done after a workout to be most effective. Stretching afterward can improve flexibility and lengthen muscles. Hold each static stretch for about 30 seconds.

Learning stretches and warm-ups specific to your exercise can also help you create a more effective workout plan. If you plan on walking a long distance, doing bodyweight deadlifts can allow you to warm up the same muscles used in walking. Touching your toes and holding after your walk will stretch the muscles that you've just worked.

Stretch until you feel a pull in your muscle, not pain. Stretching should be slightly uncomfortable instead of painful. If you're stretching too hard, the muscle can contract in an attempt to protect itself. This can lead to pain and injury. Stretch until you can feel a pull in the muscle, hold for thirty seconds, then release.

De-stress through the use of stretching. Stretching allows you to loosen muscles and release tension in any tight knots or sore areas. Improving oxygen and blood flow to the muscles and joints allows you to breathe better. Chronic stress can lead to tight muscles, especially in the face, chest, and shoulders. Stretching can help prevent these muscles from becoming tight and affecting your workout. Stretching to de-stress also makes it more enjoyable and improves your quality of life.

When you're going to work out, it's important to warm your muscles up and get them flexible and loose in order to have a more effective workout. When you're performing dynamic stretches, you're completing movements that get your muscles moving and blood flowing through your tissues. Working out then allows your muscles to operate as best as they can. When it's time to cool down, the muscles need to rest and relax. Static stretching is when you stretch a muscle and hold it for 10 - 30 seconds. This allows your muscle to stretch open and allow the blood to flow in and heal the tissues. Holding the stretch also allows you to regain control over your heart rate.

Maintaining the correct form and posture tremendously increases the benefits offered by any exercise. It is important to also remember to train all your muscle groups and divide your training plans in a way that caters to the needs of all of your body. Core training improves your balance as well as helps you with your backaches. The next few chapters are dedicated to giving you sample workout plans along with exercises addressing each muscle group specifically. In this way, you can plan your workout in ways that you enjoy doing.

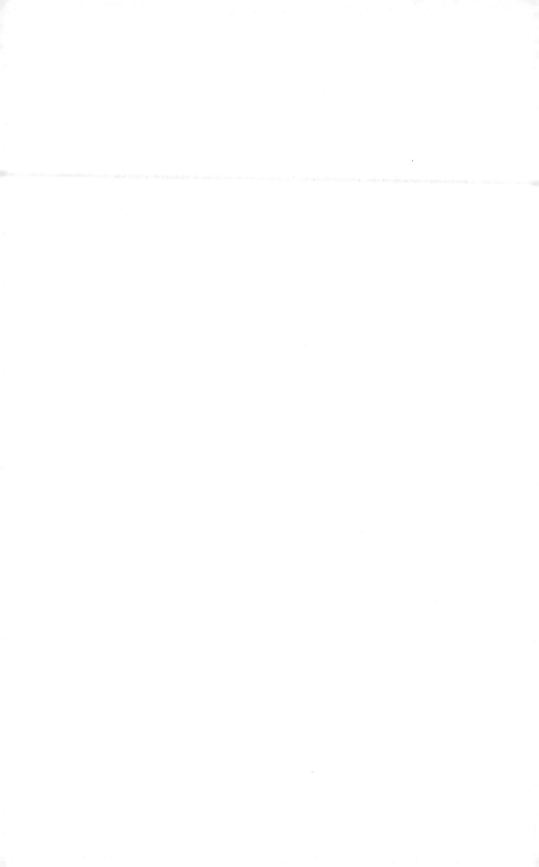

5

I HAVE A PLAN

A lot of seniors set a goal to exercise regularly for several reasons. Some of these factors, like not having time or knowledge, stand between us and our fitness goals. These barriers steal our motivation to get moving. It takes energy to push through these barriers.

Creating a workout plan removes the stress of beginning a workout plan and takes away many of the excuses that we've been using. Workout plans can be used for motivation, learning new things, and making exercise easier and more effective. A strong workout plan helps motivate you to keep going and makes it easier to build healthy habits.

Workout plans help you save time. Instead of planning each workout, you can plan for more than one workout at a time. Having a plan also helps you from forgetting certain exercises or muscle groups. If you're working towards goals, such as losing weight, improving balance, or gaining strength, missing certain muscles or exercises could put you behind in reaching your goals.

Having a workout plan also helps you track your progress. You will be able to see where you began and where you are. Maybe you started at 8 reps, now you're at 12. Making a workout plan also makes it fun! It takes the worry of what you're going to do, and how long you're going to do it out of exercising. You can focus more on your workout and less on the planning.

HOW OFTEN SHOULD I TRAIN?

An important part of a workout plan is understanding how often to train. You should train at least three times a week, but no more than six. Mixing up muscle groups and exercises can allow you to train more often. It is recommended that you do 8 – 12 reps of 50 – 80% of your max rep if you're using your weights. If your max rep is an entire gallon of milk, you'll want to do 50 – 80% of a gallon of milk each rep. It takes 6 – 8 weeks to build muscle fibers and strength. You will continue to gain these benefits for a full 20 weeks. Your ultimate goal is to set an exercise plan that you will stick with.

3-DAY SPLIT TRAINING

A 3-day split is an exercise routine that involves three training sessions per week, with a 2-day break. This could be Monday, Wednesday, Friday, or Tuesday, Thursday, and Saturday. The rest days in between allow you to recover easier, so this is the best method.

However, exercising days can be different for everyone. You can choose to work out Monday, Tuesday, Wednesday, or Tuesday, Thursday, Friday. The days you choose to exercise should fit best with your schedule. As long as you have adequate time between exercise sessions to recover, you will improve energy and muscle growth.

A 3-day workout split routine:

Improves recovery. A 3-day split rest period is much better than a 4, 5, or 6-day split. Gains take place while recovering, not during the workout.

- **Maximizes intensity.** The greater you recover, the more intense you'll be able to work out. Three days a week also allows you to have good workouts each time. Any more than three and you could miss your schedule, get burnt out, or end up stopping the program. You'll also have more power for these workouts, making them more effective.

- **Is manageable.** It is appropriate to shoot for three days of exercise a week. Exercising too much could be too imposing on your schedule. If you can't seem to find time to work out three times a week, try to look at aspects of your life and see where you can find more time.

- **Includes a variety.** Three days split program includes various schedules that you can set for yourself. You can also keep this framework throughout the year while changing the days as you need. Working out three days a week also helps you hit each of the most important muscle groups from different angles and exercises. This gives you a healthy whole-body workout.

- **Offers room for other activities.** Lifting three days a week is going to give you the energy and motivation to do the things you like. Taking the time out to exercise these three days can help you make the most of your free time.

Rest days don't mean you can't leave your bed all day. Adding flexibility and balance training during rest days can be beneficial for your goals and keeping you active.

WEEKLY WORKOUT PLAN

Now that you understand what the 3-day split training schedule is, it's time to move on to a weekly workout plan. Are you confused about which muscle groups to strength train on what days of the week? Or when should you do your balance training? Does it all seem overwhelming to you? Okay, let's simplify your workout and break it down day by day.

Mon.	Tues.	Wed.	Thurs.	Fri.	Sat.	Sun.
Chest, Shoulders, and Triceps	Balance and Flexibility Training	Legs and Core	Balance and Flexibility Training	Back and Biceps	Balance and Flexibility Training	Balance and Flexibility Training

Mon.	Tues.	Wed.	Thurs.	Fri.	Sat.	Sun.
15 Minute Walk x2	Balance and Flexibility Training	Balance and Flexibility Training	Balance and Flexibility Training	Back, Shoulders, and Biceps	30 Minutes Swimming, Cycling, or Dancing	Balance and Flexibility Training

These two plans are simply a guide. You can arrange your workouts and schedules in several ways. As long as you're resting, and including all important muscle groups, the possibilities are endless.

If you had a blank chart, what would it look like? Draw a chart and fill it in on a weekly basis. You can color code the exercises by type or after being completed. Do you normally garden on Tuesday? Maybe that should be a balance and flexibility training day. Did you forget about your granddaughter's dance recital this weekend? No problem. Simply rearrange your schedule to accommodate for rest and ensure you're not working the same groups two days in a row.

Now that you have learned what workouts you can do and how to schedule them, you are all set to learn how to do your workouts. The next chapters will teach you how to perform exercises step by step. Don't give up now, you've got this.

6

UPPER BODY EXERCISES

Upper body exercises combine active movements of your core and shoulders with deep breathing exercises. Make sure to inhale through your nose and see that your belly button rises then you exhale through your mouth thus lowering your belly button. These exercises help with the ventilation of your lungs along with improving posture, rib mobility, and flexibility of the upper chest. This chapter will suggest a list of chest exercises that you can do along with pictures to understand the proper form of each step.

WHAT YOU NEED

As we've discussed earlier, household items can be used for your workout requirements. A few items you can use to improve your workout are:

- **A kitchen chair.** Chairs with no armrests are great to keep close by when working out. This will give you the confidence you need to keep going. Plus, you can sit or rest when you need it.
- **A counter.** Using a counter to hold onto while you're doing your exercises can provide you with safety and stability. You can focus more on the muscles you're working and your form.
- **Painter's tape.** Walking exercises can be done by walking in a straight line. This can be hard for some seniors to do. To motivate you to keep going, take a long piece of painter's tape, or masking tape, and place it on the ground as straight as you can. You can ask someone to help you put it down, so it's as straight as possible.
- **Arm and ankle weights.** These weights are a great way to add a little resistance to your normal activities or exercises. You'll want to stay below 2 pounds on each arm or ankle. More weight than this can cause a strain on certain joints.
- **A paper with writing**. Reading and walking can be challenging for some adults. It can affect balance and lead to dizziness. Working on reading and walking can help you in the grocery store or at the doctor's office. You can start by holding onto the wall or counter and taking a few steps at a time while reading.

When working out, it's important to avoid tacky or rubber shoes. This type of shoe can cause you to get caught up on rugs or other flooring. Wearing a smooth bottom shoe, such as a dancing shoe, can allow you to walk without any catches. Also, be sure to clear any objects that you may trip over. Slippers, dog toys, or decorations on the floor can cause you to interrupt your exercise to step over them or move them.

Warm-Up Exercises

Warm-up exercises are important for preparing your muscles to work. Warmups should be more than just a few stretches. You should also warm up the heart and lungs. A good warmup increases blood flow, improves muscle reaction time, and mentally prepares you for the workout. Working out without warming up first can lead to injury. Check out this list of warm-up exercises and how to do them below.

Shoulder rolls.

1. Stand (or sit) up straight, look straight ahead, and rest your arms at your side.

2. Lift your shoulders up to your ears then roll them into a full circle.

    a. Keep your torso as still as you can. Focus on using the muscles in your shoulders to lift and roll them.

3. Do 20 circles as large as you can go.

4. Then, roll your shoulders 20 circles in the opposite direction.

Shoulder Rolls

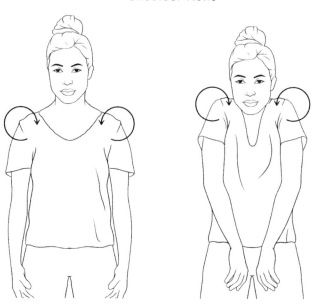

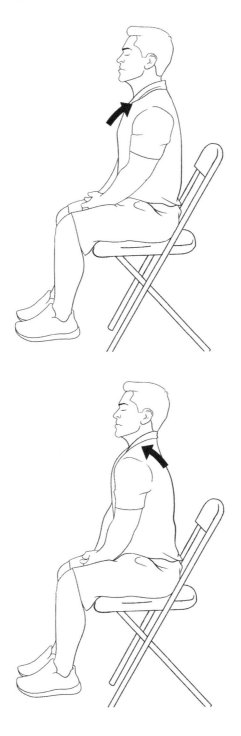

Shoulder squeezes.

1. Stand (or sit) up straight and rest your arms at your side.

2. Bend your arms at the elbow in a 90-degree angle.

3. Slowly swing your elbows behind you, keeping them bent (as if you're skiing).

4. Squeeze your shoulder blades together. (Pretend as if you're trying to touch your elbows together, behind your back).

5. Try to bring your arms back at the same time, aiming for a symmetrical squeeze.

6. Perform 1 – 2 sets of 10 – 20 reps.

Shoulder Squeeze

Neck stretches.

1. Stand (or sit) up straight and rest your arms at your side.

2. Tilt your head back as far as you can comfortably. Be sure to have hold onto something for balance and stop if you feel pain or if you're about to fall.

3. Slowly lower your chin down to your chest. Make sure you're breathing and if you feel dizzy, pause for a few minutes. You should feel a pull in the back of your neck.

4. Look up, then down 10 – 15 times.

5. Look left, then right 10 – 15 times.

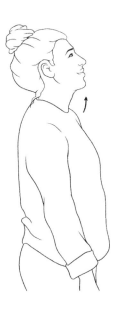

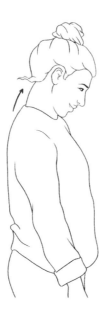

Leg swings.

1. Stand and rest your hand on a wall, table, counter, or chair for stability.

2. With your feet shoulder-width apart, take the right leg and swing it in front of you as if you're kicking a ball. Raise your leg as high as you can without moving the opposite side of your body or losing balance. Lower it back to the ground, swinging it backwards if you can.

3. Repeat for 10 – 15 reps.

4. Turn around, grab your stability tool, and repeat with the other leg.

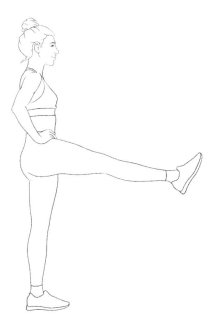

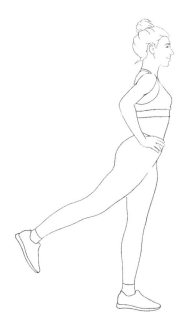

Seated ankle curls.

1. Set up straight in a chair.

2. Take your right leg and cross it over the left or extend it in front of you and raise it off the ground a few inches.

3. Roll your ankle in circles, making big circles with your toes. This movement may feel jerky. Keep your leg as still as you can and make the circles as smooth as possible.

4. Do 10 circles one way, then 10 circles another way.

* To make this more challenging, raise both legs and circle both ankles at the same time.

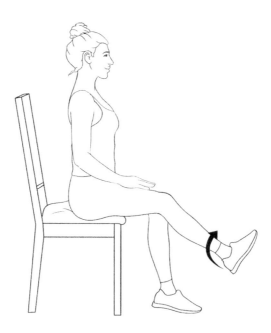

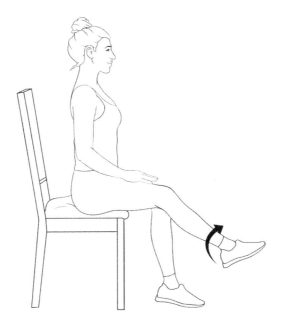

Sitting hamstring stretch.

1. Sit up in a chair with feet shoulder-width apart and flat on the ground. Scoot towards the front of the seat.

2. Stretch out your right leg, leaving your heel on the floor.

3. Place your hands on your thighs, palm down, and reach towards your knees. Keep your back straight and lean forward at the hip. Be sure not to topple forward.

4. Stop when you feel a stretch in the back of your thigh. If you notice your knee is painful or being stretched, bend it a little.

5. Hold the stretch for about 20 seconds.

6. Repeat on the other side.

* You can lean deeper into the stretch during the 20-second count

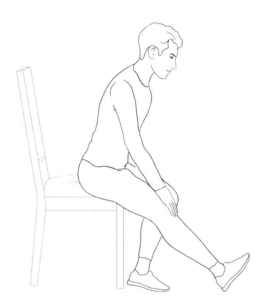

Seated shin stretch.

1. Sit in a chair and cross your left ankle over your right. Keep your right foot flat on the floor.

2. Curl the toes on your left foot and squeeze your legs together. You should feel the stretch on the muscles on the front of the calf, around the long, thin, hard shin bone.

3. Hold for 20 seconds, then repeat on the other foot.

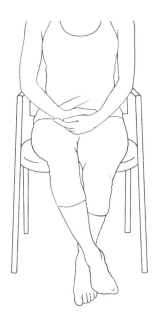

Seated hip lifts.

1. Sit up in the chair and rest your back against it.

2. Hold the sides of the chair and raise your right foot off the floor and your right hip off the seat.

3. Hold it for 10 – 20 seconds, then lower it back onto the seat. Repeat 3 times on each side.

* To adjust the exercise, you can cross your legs and lift the hip of the top leg. You can also slide to the front part of the chair.

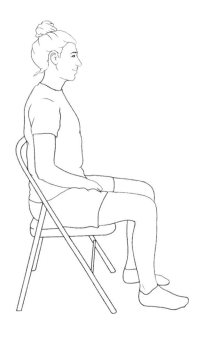

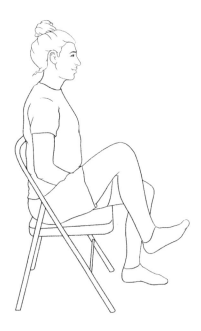

You should warm up your entire body, even if you're only working on parts of it.

Upper Body Stretching Exercises

Strength training is beneficial for the muscles in many ways. However, flexibility is just as important for muscles. With these strength exercises, it's time for you to learn about upper body flexibility exercises.

Shoulder and Upper Back Stretch

1. Press your hands together in a prayer motion. Take a deep breath through the nose, and exhale as you reach your arms high into the sky. (Think again about the "Y" movement in YMCA).

2. Lower your arms back to your side.

3. Repeat for 10 reps.

* Keep your forearms together as you raise your arms. Keep your chest up and squeeze your shoulder blades when lowering your arms.

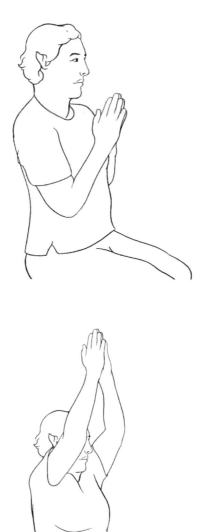

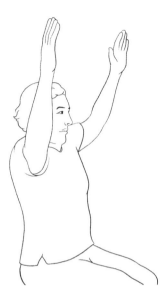

Neck Side Stretch

1. Sit comfortably in a chair.

2. Reach your right hand behind your back and lean against it. Your hand should be snug between your back and the chair. Take your left hand and place it on the top of your head.

3. Pull your head to the side, keeping your face straight forward. Pull down your head until you feel a stretch in the side of your neck. Hold for 5 seconds, then release.

4. Repeat on the other side.

* Be sure not to pull too hard and stop if you get dizzy. Breathe normally. If you've had a stroke in the past, do not hold the stretch longer than 2 – 3 seconds.

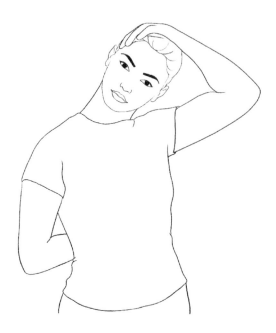

Neck Rotation

1. Sit comfortably.

2. Look to the left as far as you can and hold for 5 seconds.

3. Look to the right for 5 seconds.

4. Bring your left ear to your left shoulder and hold for 5 seconds.

5. Bring your right ear to your right shoulder and hold for 5 seconds.

6. Return to normal position.

* Breathe normally. Stop if there's pain or dizziness. Stretch your ear to your shoulder. Don't bring your shoulder to your ear. This gives you a better stretch. To improve balance, do this standing up.

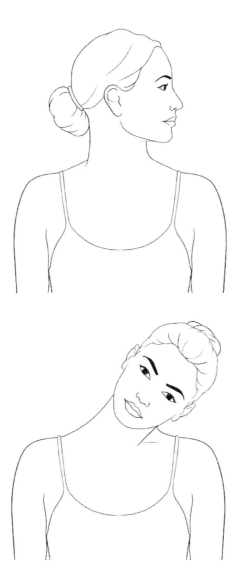

Shoulder Circles

1. Sit in a chair.

2. Reach up and rest your fingertips on your shoulders. Breathe normally.

3. Roll your shoulders 15 times forward, then 15 times backward.

*Imagine you're drawing circles with your elbows. Keep your ribs and elbows high.

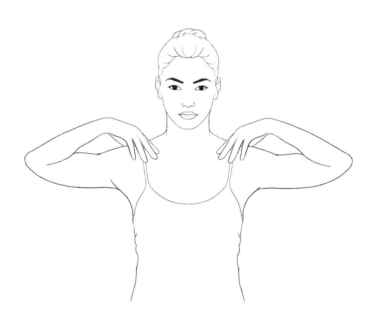

Shoulder Stretch

1. Sit or stand comfortably.

2. Bring your right hand over to your left shoulder. (Like you're patting yourself on the back.)

3. Grasp your right elbow with your left hand.

4. Pull your elbow towards your shoulder and hold for 10 – 15 seconds.

5. Repeat on the other side.

* Breathe normally: in through the nose and out through the mouth. Stop if there's pain or dizziness. To make it more of a challenge, hold the stretch longer or keep your elbow straight when moving it back towards the shoulder.

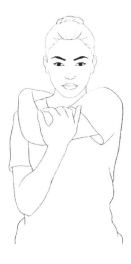

Chest Stretch

1. Sit in a chair.

2. Put your hands behind your head.

3. Inhale as you stretch your hands back, opening your chest and spreading it forward.

4. Exhale as you bring your arms down.

5. Repeat 3 times

* Keep ribs lifted when you breathe in and bring the neck and shoulders back. For an increase in intensity, lean to the left and breathe out, then to the right and breathe out, while you have your hands behind your head.

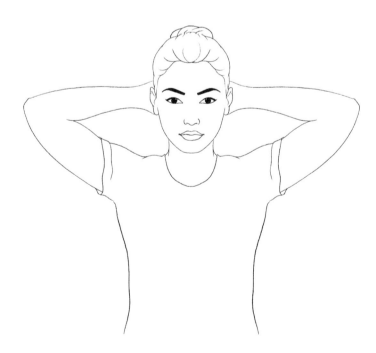

Overhead Reach

1. Sit comfortably, interlace your fingers, place them in your lap, and take a deep breath.

2. Keeping your fingers together, raise your hands high into the sky. (Like you're making a big "O".)

3. Lower your hands.

4. Repeat 10 times.

* Breathe in while moving your hands up, then breathe out while moving your hands down. Sit straight up and keep your ribs lifted. To take it up a notch, lean to the left while you have your hands over your head. Lean back to the middle, then lower them. Repeat with your right side on the next lift.

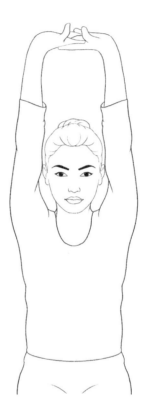

Reach Back

1. Stand with a chair behind you. Interlace your fingers behind your back as you take a deep breath through the nose.

2. Breathe out and gently push your arms back. Pause for a few seconds, then return to the beginning position.

3. Repeat 10 times.

* Keep your spine straight and stop if there's pain. To make it harder, lean forward at your waist and exhale when you bring your arms back.

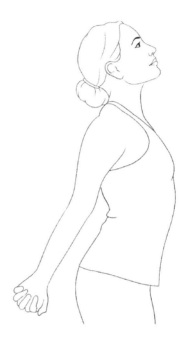

Tricep Stretch

1. Sit in a chair with your left arm and palm facing up.

2. Bring your left arm over your head and pat yourself on the back. (Nice job!)

3. Grab your left elbow with your right hand and push it backwards. You should feel your left hand moving down your back.

4. Release after 10 – 15 seconds. Repeat on the other arm.

* Breathe in through the nose and out through the mouth. Stop if there's pain and don't push so hard that you put stress on your shoulder joint. If you're looking for more of a challenge, raise your right elbow as you're pressing your left elbow. Moving both up will deepen the stretch.

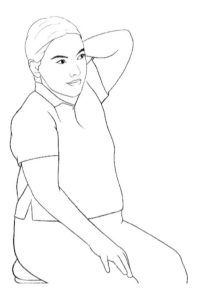

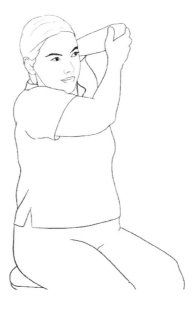

Hand Stretch

1. Float your arms straight in front of you with your palms facing down.

2. Open and close your hand, spreading your fingers as wide as you can in between.

3. Repeat 10 times.

* Breathe normally. Don't strain or attempt to squeeze hard. If your shoulders get tired of upholding your hands, rest them in your lap. To improve effectiveness, do wrist circles while opening and closing the hands.

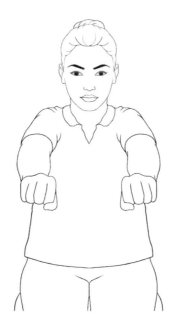

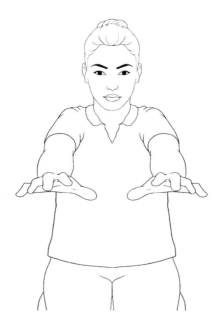

Arm Raises

1. Stand comfortably with your arms at your sides. Lift your ribs and relax your shoulders.

2. Inhale while lifting your arms straight out and above your head. (Keep your arms straight, think of a field goal in football.)

3. Repeat this 10 times.

*Breathe in while you're moving your arms up, breathe out while you're lowering them. Don't arch your back and be sure to keep your fingers open and hands loose. With each reach, try to get closer and closer to the sky or ceiling. You can do this against a wall for posture alignment.

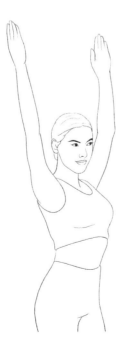

Strength Training the Upper Body

Strength training is the process of loading the muscle with more weight than it is used to, to promote strength and build muscles. Here is a list of strength training exercises that target the upper body:

Overhead press.

1. Sit or stand with your feet shoulder-width apart.

2. Hold your homemade weights in each hand even with your chest, with your palms facing forward.

3. Raise your hands into the air, pressing the weights up.

4. Lower your arms to the starting position and repeat 10 times for 1 – 2 sets.

* Inhale while pushing up, exhale while lowering down. Sit down if there is stress on your back. Keep your chest up and facing out and avoid arching your back.

** To increase the intensity, place one foot in front of the other and lunge forward while lifting the weights straight up.

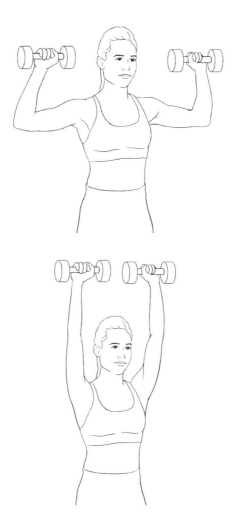

Bicep curls.

1. Hold your water bottles in your hands, down by your side, with your palms facing out. Keep your shoulders back and your chest up and out.

2. Bend your arm at the elbow and raise the water bottle to your chest. Inhale while moving upward, exhale when lowering down.

3. Lower back to your side.

4. Repeat 10 times for 1-2 sets on each arm.

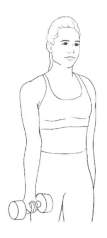

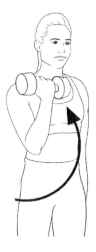

Overhead elbow extension.

1. Hold your creative weights with your palm facing inward. You can sit or stand.

2. To get into position, raise your weight to your ear then push back a few inches, pointing your elbow up. Your hand should be hanging a little behind your shoulder.

3. Extend your arm straight up, then bring it back down to position. Inhale while raising, exhale while lowering.

4. Repeat on each arm 10 times.

* You can hold the elbow of the arm you're exercising with your opposite hand for support if needed. Sit in a chair with a back if you feel a strain in your back. Try holding at the top for about ten seconds if you want to make it harder.

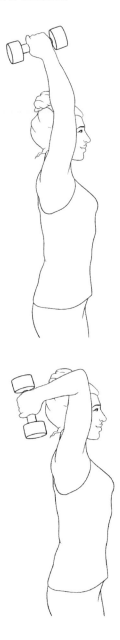

Triceps Kickbacks

1. If sitting, lean over your knee so your arm has room to extend. If standing, hold onto something for support and lean forward, moving the hips back. You can bend the knees.

2. Hang your arm down in front of you, with your weight in hand.

3. Bend your elbow up to your side. Reach back as far as you can. (Think of swinging your arm back before throwing a bowling ball). Keep your body and elbow still and use a slow, moderate speed. Don't throw or swing them. Exhale while pushing back, inhale while returning to starting position.

4. Return to resting position. Complete 10 reps on each side.

* To make it harder, perform 20 reps or hold for about 10 seconds once you've reached behind you.

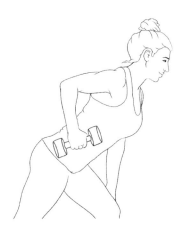

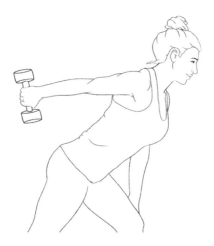

Diagonal Inward Shoulder Raise

1. Sit or stand with the weight in your hand, and palm facing out.

2. Slowly swing your hand in a diagonal motion across your chest and towards your opposite shoulder. Breathe while lifting your hand across. Exhale while lowering it.

3. Repeat this motion 10 times then switch to your other arm.

* Keep a slow, comfortable pace. If it becomes painful during the end of your arm movement, only lift in the pain-free range. To increase the intensity, stand, use a heavier weight, or do 20 repetitions.

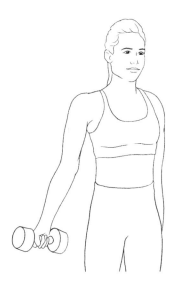

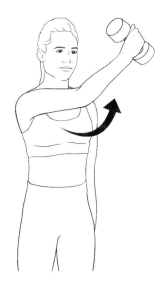

Diagonal Outward Shoulder Raise

1. Sit or stand with your handmade weight in your left hand.

2. Reach the hand over to the right hip. (Imagine buckling in your seatbelt but keeping your upper body straight.)

3. Raise your hand from your hip and swing it up and out to the left, in a diagonal motion. (The same movement as the "Y" in the YMCA song). Inhale while bringing the weight up. Exhale while lowering it down.

4. Return to the resting position.

5. Repeat on each side for 10 reps.

* Hold your weight tight enough so that you don't throw it, but don't squeeze. Maintain your posture and stay below 2 pounds if you have shoulder issues.

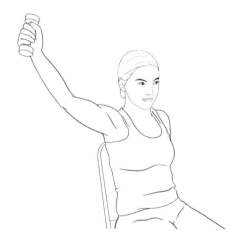

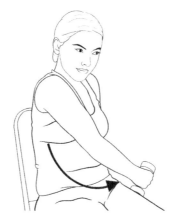

Shoulder Shrugs

1. Stand or sit with your water bottles in hand. Make sure your arms can hang freely at your side.

2. Slowly shrug your shoulders. (As if you're gesturing 'I don't know'.) Inhale as you raise them, exhale as you lower them.

3. Do 10 – 15 reps.

* Breathe out as you bring your back and shoulders up. Focus on lifting your ribcage. Try to keep your elbows straight and shrug as high as you comfortably can. To add intensity, try standing up or doing 20 repetitions.

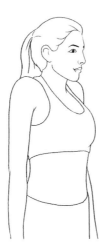

Shoulder Press Lying Down

1. Lie on your back on a comfortable, flat surface. Make sure your head, torso, and behind are flat.

2. Bend your arms with your weights to a 90-degree angle. Push your hands to the ceiling with your palms facing together. Inhale as you push up, exhale as you lower them.

3. Lower them back to position. Be mindful not to drop them or let your elbows slam onto the floor. Have a gentle and controlled motion from start to finish.

4. Repeat 10 times

* Make sure you're able to get up or have help from someone before getting into the floor for this exercise. Use light to medium size weights. Keep forearms parallel and move weights until your elbow is fully extended. To make it more challenging, raise your shoulders off the ground when you're pushing the weights up.

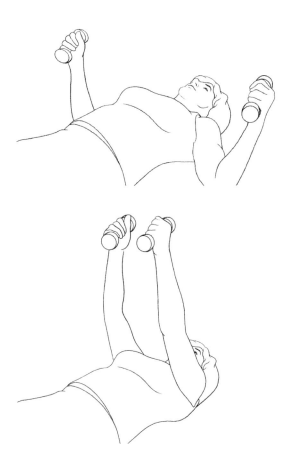

Upright Rows

1. Start by standing with your weights in front of your hips. Your feet should be shoulder-width apart.

2. Make sure both palms are facing you and raise both weights to your chin. You should feel this in your shoulders. Inhale as you raise the weight, exhale as you lower it. Keep your palms facing you and your elbows pointing out. You will lift the weight straight up to your chin.

3. Lower the weight to the starting area.

4. Repeat for a total of 10 times.

* Keep the back straight and shoulders down. This exercise is best when standing. To make it harder, stand with one foot in front of the other, use a heavier weight, or do 15 – 20 reps.

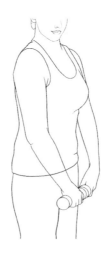

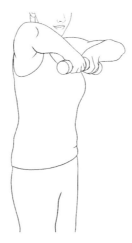

Bent Over Rows

1. Stand with your hand on a support system, such as a wall or cane. Let your hand and weight dangle down.

2. Lift the weight to your chest, making sure the elbow points backwards. Inhale as you bring the weight up. Exhale as you lower it.

3. Return to the starting positions.

4. Repeat 10 times on each arm.

* Keep shoulders and back even. Keep the elbow next to the ribs. To elevate it, bring the weight to touch the ribcage and hold for 10 seconds.

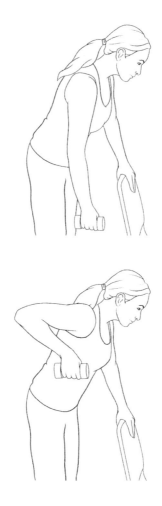

Side Shoulder Raise

1. Stand with your elbow straight, palm facing forward, and arm against your side.

2. Reach out to the side and up above your head. Keep your arm straight. (Think of the Statue of Liberty). Breathe out when reaching up. Breathe in when lowering your hand down.

3. Return to resting position.

4. Repeat for 10 – 15 reps on each side.

* Keep your elbows slightly flexed. Control your arms as you lower them to your side.

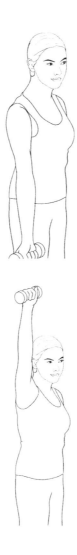

Elbow Side Extensions

1. Stand with your feet shoulder-width apart. Hold your weights to your chest with your elbows bent and pointing outwards.

2. Stretch your arms out to each side, opening your chest wide. Keep your arms up, as in a "T" position. Breathe in while spreading your arms, breathe out while bringing them back in.

3. Fold your arms back to return to the resting position.

4. Repeat 10 – 12 times.

* Keep your elbows at chest level. Keep your upper body straight and facing forward. To make it harder, stand with one foot in front of the other. Lunge forward as you extend the weights on both sides.

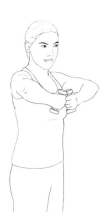

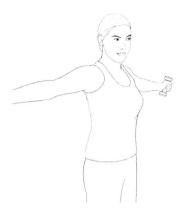

Modified Skull Crushers

1. Lie back in a chair with your legs stretched in front of you. You can cross them at the ankle.

2. With your weights in hand, reach up and behind your head, keeping your elbows in.

3. Extend your arms at the elbow straight up. Breathe in while extending your arms, breathe out while bringing them back.

4. Keeping your shoulders and elbows still, lower them back down behind your head, in the resting position.

5. Repeat for 10 – 15 reps.

* Keep your back strong and use only your arms. Be cautious not to slide out of your chair. To increase the intensity, do 20 reps, or hold for 10 seconds at the top of the exercise.

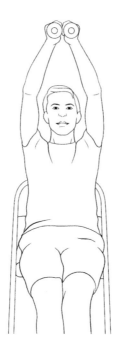

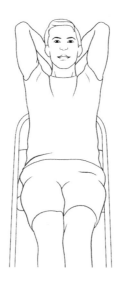

Forward Punches

1. Take your weights in your hand and hold them in front of you, as if you are in a fighting stance. Make sure your posture is strong.

2. Slowly punch one arm out and bring it back to the chest.

3. Repeat with the other arm.

4. Do a total of 10 reps on each side.

* Breathe out while punching out, breathe in while bringing the weights back. You can lean slightly to each side when you punch. To make it more exciting, increase the weight or double the number of reps.

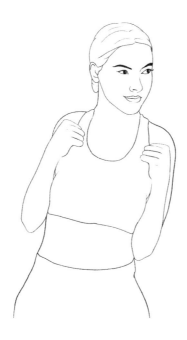

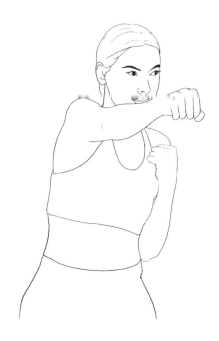

Reverse Fly

1. Stand, or sit in a chair with your feet flat on the ground and together.

2. Lean over slightly, letting your arms fall in front of you.

3. With a weight in each hand, lift your arms out to the sides, focusing on squeezing your shoulder blades together. Exhale as you reach out, inhale as you bring them down.

4. Repeat 10 times

* Keep your back straight. Use slow and controlled move-ment. Avoid throwing your arms and make sure you're breath-

ing. Double the reps or hold for 10 seconds when you get to the back to make it harder.

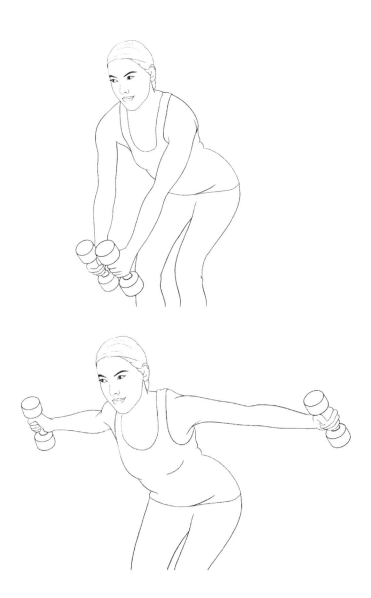

Lateral Raises

1. Sit or stand and have a homemade weight in each hand.

2. Bend your arms at a 90-degree angle with your elbows near your hips and your weights on the outside of each knee.

3. Raise your arms up without extending your arm. (Think of the chicken dance, except your hands fly out with your elbows). Exhale as you raise your arms, inhale as you lower them.

4. Repeat 10 times

* Keep your arms bent and focus on sitting up straight. Keep your chest out and your head up. To make it harder, hold at the top for 10 seconds. You can also stop once you've raised your arms, stretch them out, bring them back, then lower them down.

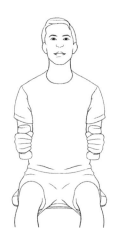

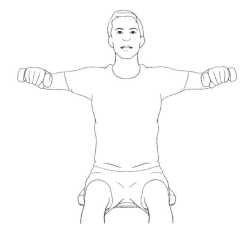

Single Arm Overhead Triceps

1. Take one weighted bottle and raise it straight up above your head.

2. Keeping your elbow still, only moving your forearm and hand, lower the weight back down and touch it on the back of your shoulder.

3. You should feel the burn in your upper arm on both sides.

Repeat on each side for 10 reps.

*Be cautious not to hit yourself in the head with your weight. If it hurts your elbow, don't stretch it completely out. To make this more intense, stand with one leg in front of the other, or do both arms at the same time.

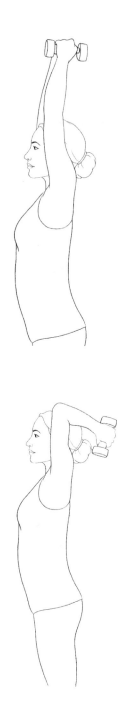

Static Stretching

It's important to stretch and take a few minutes to relax after a workout before returning to daily activities. Static stretches are a great way to cool down the muscles and allow them to return to normal activity. You're going to want to perform these stretches after exercising.

Look Ups

1. Sit comfortably with your hands in your lap or on armrests.

2. Look up as high as you can. Ideally, look directly up at the ceiling.

3. Hold this stretch for about 20 – 30 seconds.

* Breathe in through the nose and out through the mouth. Stop if you feel pain or dizziness.

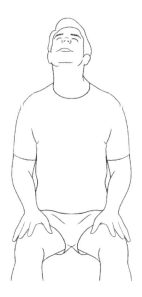

Chest Open Stretches

1. Spread your arms wide in front of you.

2. Open your hands and face them out.

3. Hold this for 20 – 30 seconds.

4. Squeeze your shoulder blades together and let your arms fall a little, focusing on that pull in the shoulder blades.

5. Hold this for 15 seconds.

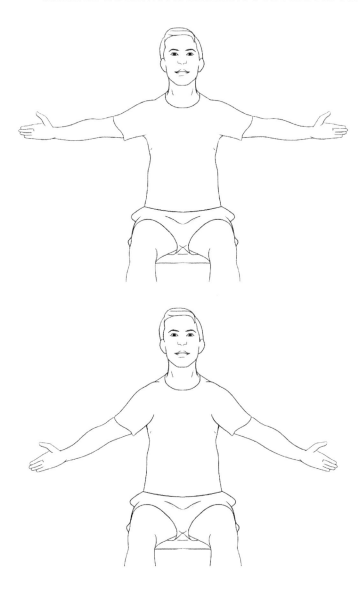

Spine Stretch

1. Sit or stand comfortably.

2. Interlace your fingers and point both palms away from you.

3. Raise your arms high above your head, pressing your palms out gently.

4. Hold for 30 seconds.

5. Return to rest.

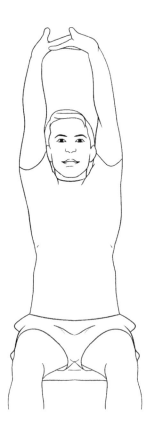

Lower Back Stretch

1. Sit up straight in a chair and scoot to the edge.

2. Reach behind you and place your hands on your lower back.

3. Push your elbows into the back of your seat and lean into your hands.

4. Slightly lean back, you should feel the stretch in your back.

5. Hold for 15 seconds.

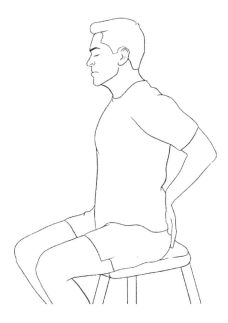

Shake out your arms and legs and take a deep breath. You've just completed a full upper body strength, balance, and flexibility program! How exciting! The upper body exercises are aimed at improving the range of motion of your shoulders and upper back with these stretching and strength training exercises. The next chapter tells you about the lower body strengthening and stretching exercises to help you with the movability and flexibility of your ankles, hips, and thighs.

7

LOWER BODY EXERCISES

Strength exercises for your legs will help you to easily stand from a chair, climb steps, side-stepping around obstacles in your way and all your ADLs (activities of daily living) like bathing, cooking, cleaning, etc. Training your legs will help you gain an improved balance. It will also enhance the power, coordination, and overall range of motion in your lower body.

Remember to always warm up. We covered some of the best warmups in the last chapter, so feel free to use those! It's important to warm up before working out legs because they carry most of our movements. There are many benefits to training the lower body. Training the lower limbs can:

- Improve bone strength
- Improve balance

- Boost stamina
- Boost confidence
- Reduce the risk of falling
- Reduces physical weakness
- Lowers levels of pain
- Reduces hip injuries
- Decrease knee injuries
- Improved stability
- Increased energy
- Improve dexterity and balance

Stretching is a very important part of exercising. Stretching your muscles allows them to be more flexible. Having flexible muscles allows you to get more effective workouts. Here are some stretches that are sure to elevate your workout.

Seated Lifts

1. Grab either side of a chair for support while sitting.

2. Raise your right hip off the chair and hold for 10 – 20 seconds.

3. Shift to the other hip and lift and hold for 10 – 20 seconds.

* Breathe normally, in through the nose and out through the mouth. Be cautious if you've recently had a hip replacement. Leave your back against the chair. If you need to, hold your knee up. For more of a stretch, scoot to the edge of the seat and twist when you raise.

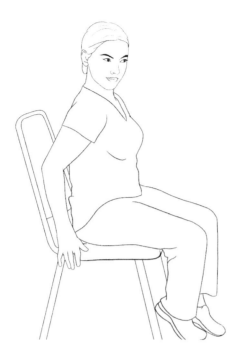

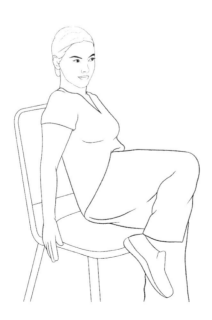

Standing Quadriceps Stretch

1. Stand while holding something for support.

2. Grasp your right ankle behind you and pull it to your buttocks.

3. Hold for 10 – 20 seconds then repeat with the other leg.

* Breathe normally, in through the nose and out through the mouth. Stop if you feel pain in your knees or ankle. Grab your pant leg if that is easier to hold. Don't pull too hard. Look straight ahead and hold for 30 seconds to improve outcomes.

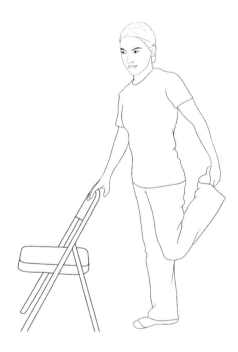

Back Stretch

1. Stand with feet shoulder-width apart.

2. Put your hands on your hips and place your palms against your bottom. Breathe in through your nose.

3. Arch your spine back and hold for 10 seconds. Repeat 3 times.

* Don't overextend. If there's pain in your spine then stop. Don't tilt the head back too far. To make it harder, place one foot in front of the other.

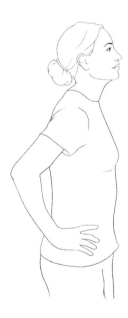

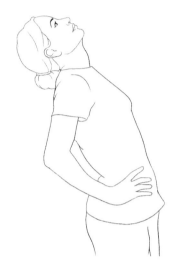

Inner Thigh Stretch

1. Stand while holding something for support.

2. Place your feet far apart, be careful not to lose your balance or put yourself in an uncomfortable position.

3. Bend down, and point your knees and toes outward at 45 degrees. You'll feel this in your inner thigh.

4. Return to a standing position.

5. Hold for 10 – 20 seconds and repeat 3 times total.

* Breathe normally, in the nose and out the mouth. Keep your torso upright. To improve balance, hold your arms out on either side of you.

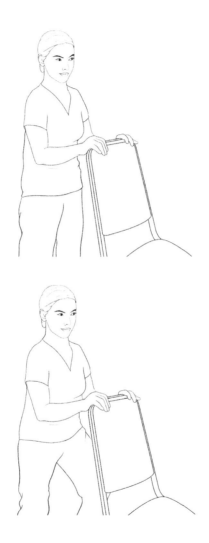

Calf Stretch

1. Face a wall and place both hands on it in front of your face, palm down.

2. Place the toes of your right foot against the wall.

3. Lean your hips toward the wall, leaving your left foot flat on the floor.

4. Hold for 10 – 20 seconds. Switch sides.

* If you have pain, stop, and try it again while staying in your pain-free range of motion. Breathe normally and keep the back straight. To improve balance, use only one hand on the wall or place them on your hips.

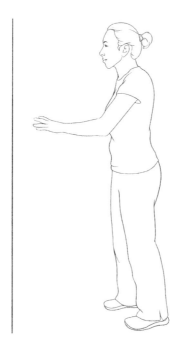

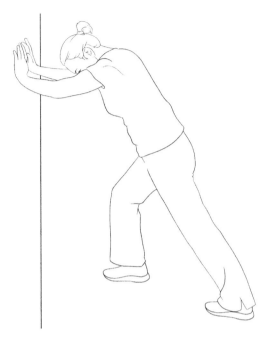

Hip Side Stretch

1. Stand about a foot away from the wall. Place your right hand on the wall for stability.

2. Cross your left leg over your right leg.

3. Lean your right hip towards the wall until you feel a stretch.

4. Hold for 10 – 20 seconds then switch to the other leg.

* Breathe normally. If you have knee or hip pain, ease up on the stretch. Only lean your hips into the wall. Leave your upper body upright. You can take a small step when crossing your legs. Hold for longer or do 2 – 3 sets on each side for improved results.

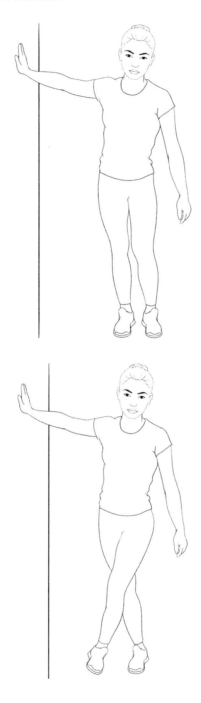

Hip Rotation Stretch

1. Sit comfortably.

2. Rest your left ankle on your right knee.

3. Press down onto your knee until you feel the stretch.

4. Hold for 10 – 20 seconds then repeat with the other leg.

*Breathe normally. If you cannot rest your ankle on your knee, simply cross your ankles and push your knee down and out. Be cautious if you've just had hip or knee surgery. You can lean forward to increase the stretch.

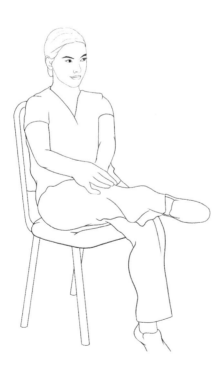

Soleus Stretch

1. Face a wall.

2. Place your right foot in front of your left. Put your palms on the wall for support.

3. Bend your knees until you feel a stretch.

4. Keep your heels on the ground and hold for 10 – 20 seconds.

5. Switch legs then repeat.

*Breathe in through the nose and out through the mouth. Keep yourself upright as you lower yourself. Stop if you feel pain. Hold the position for 30 seconds to make it more advanced.

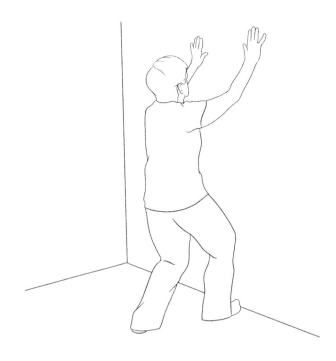

Hamstring Stretch

1. Place your left leg out flat on the surface while your right foot rests on the ground. You can lay your left leg on a bed, couch, or chair that's even with your hip and allows you to stretch your leg out.

2. Lean forward and reach for your left ankle, knee, or thigh. Lean as far as you're comfortable.

3. Hold for 10 – 20 seconds and repeat with the opposite leg.

* Breathe in through the nose and out through the mouth. Try to sit upright and lean over at the hips. To deepen the stretch, wrap a towel under your foot and pull yourself towards your foot.

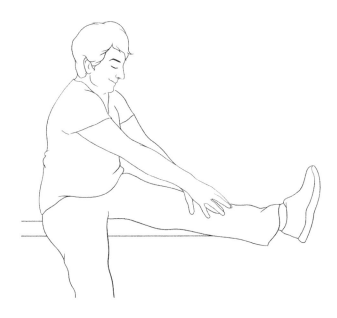

Knee to Chest

1. Sit comfortably in a chair.

2. Raise your knee up and hold it with your hands, hugging your knee to your chest.

3. Hold for 10 – 20 seconds then return your leg to the floor.

4. Repeat on the other leg.

* Breathe normally. Make sure you're not pulling too hard. If you feel pain in the knee, unbend the knee a little. Grab the ankle or shin for a deeper stretch.

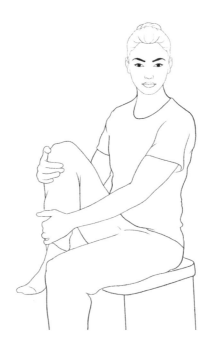

Ankle Stretch

1. Sit on the edge of a chair. Make sure there is nothing under the chair.

2. Tuck your right foot under the chair with your toes pointed down and touching the ground.

3. Push on the foot until you feel a stretch.

4. Hold for 20 – 30 seconds for each ankle.

* Hold the sides of the chair for support. To stretch the thigh further, move the foot on the outside of the chair and let the knee dip lower.

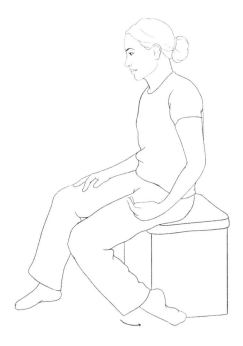

Strength Training Exercises

Ankle Circles

1. Sit in a chair and leave your foot flat on the ground.

2. Extend your right leg in front of you and roll your ankle 2o times. Imagine drawing circles with your toes.

3. Roll your ankle in the opposite direction 20 times.

4. Repeat on the other side.

* Breathe normally. It's normal for your ankle to pop when rolling. If there is pain then stop.

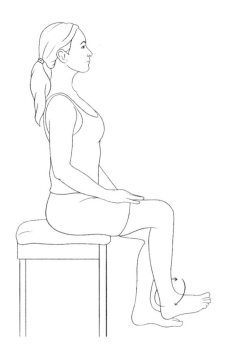

Hip Marching

1. Sit up with your feet flat on the ground.

2. Place your hands on your knees.

3. Raise your right knee as high as you can.

4. Lower your leg, then repeat with the other. Continue for a total of 10 reps each.

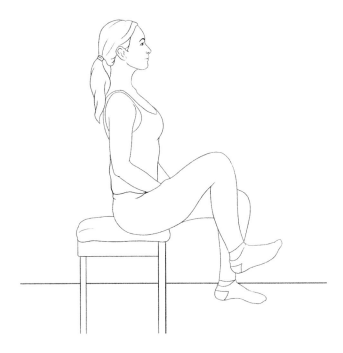

Knee Extension

1. Sit up with your feet flat on the ground.

2. Straighten your leg in front of you, extending your leg as far as you can, comfortably. Inhale when raising your leg, and exhale while lowering it.

3. Return your foot to the ground. Hold onto the chair for support.

4. Repeat with the other leg and continue for a total of 10 reps on each leg.

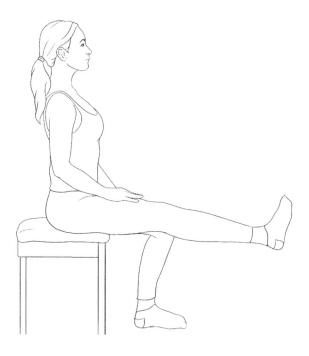

* Move slowly without jerking your leg or kicking. Tilt your toes back towards your body. To make it more challenging, add ankle weights.

Calf Raises

1. Stand up holding a chair or wall to balance yourself.

2. Press yourself up on the tip of your toes. (Like you're trying to look over something.)

3. Press yourself up then down for 10 reps.

* Breathe in as you push up and exhale as you push out. Keep your feet a few inches apart for balance. Add weights to make it more effective.

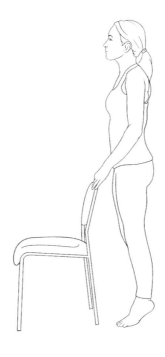

Standing Knee Flexion

1. Stand up holding a chair or wall to balance yourself.

2. Bend your knee as far as you can without pain.

3. Squeeze at the top, then lower it down.

4. Repeat on each leg for 10 reps.

* Breathe in as you raise the leg, and exhale as you lower the leg back down. Keep the movements slow and controlled. Be cautious not to kick whatever you're using to balance yourself. Add ankle weights to make the thighs stronger.

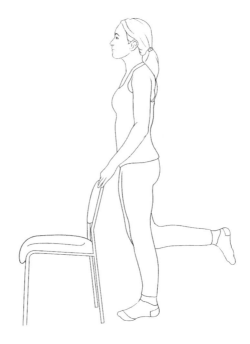

Side Hip Raises

1. Stand up holding a counter or cane to balance yourself.

2. Raise your right leg out beside you as high as you can.

3. Return to the ground. Repeat for 10 times on each side.

* Breathe in as you're raising your leg out, then breathe out and you're bringing it back down. Be aware not to kick anything (or anyone) beside you. Work on keeping your leg straight as you move it out. Add ankle weights to make it more difficult.

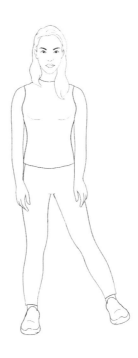

Sit to Stand

1. Start with a chair behind you and your knees about two inches in front of the seat.

2. Hold your hands out in front of you with your palms down.

3. Slowly lean forward at your hips and squat to sit in the chair. Before you touch the chair, pause, and rise back to a standing position. Breathe in as you squat down and breathe out as you stand up.

4. Repeat for 10 – 12 reps.

* Make sure your knees are shoulder width apart and they aren't buckling or moving towards one another when sitting down. Focus on putting extra weight in your heels. Hold your gallon jug of sand or water against your chest to increase benefits.

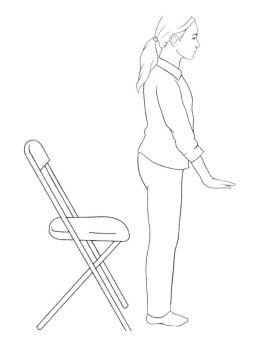

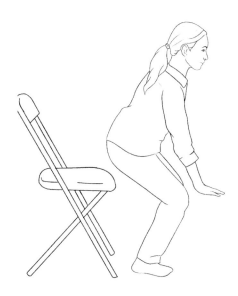

Heel Stand

1. Stand up holding a counter or chair to balance yourself.

2. Raise your toes and the balls of your feet up to the ceiling, shifting all of your weight onto your heels.

3. Lower your toes flat to the ground.

4. Repeat for 10 – 12 reps.

* Breathe in as you raise your toes and breathe out as you lay them down. Double the reps to make it more difficult.

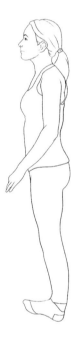

Lunges

1. Stand with your feet shoulder-width apart. You can put your hands on your waist or stretched out on either side to improve stability.

2. Step forward with your right leg, while keeping your upper body upright and your left foot on the floor.

3. Bend your right leg, as if you are picking something up, but don't lean over. Don't bend the knee too far.

4. Hold it for a second, then step back into a standing position.

5. Repeat for 10 reps on each side.

* Breathe out as you're stepping forward, then inhale when stepping backwards. Start by taking a small step away from the other leg. Increase distance in your step as you feel more comfortable with the distance. Keep a chair close to grab in case you need to rest. Hold weights or increase reps to take it up a notch.

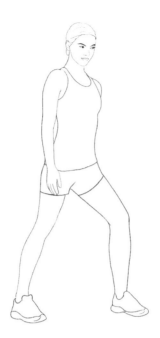

Straight Leg Raise

1. Lie on your back. Bend your left leg and place your foot flat on the floor. Leave your right leg laid out.

2. Lay your hands flat on the floor beside you. Keep your right leg straight and raise it up until your knees are side-by-side.

3. Return the leg to the ground. Repeat on the other side for 10 reps each.

* Inhale as you raise your leg and exhale as you lower your leg. Don't let your knee raise past your other knee. Hold the knees together for 10 seconds to make the exercise more challenging.

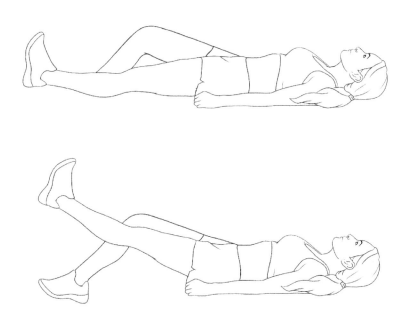

Partial Squats

1. Stand up holding a chair or wall to balance yourself.

2. Bend your knees and lower your body as far as you're comfortable with.

3. Return to a standing position.

4. Repeat for 10 – 15 reps.

* Breathe in while moving up and exhale while moving down. Look forward and keep your heels on the ground. Hold weights for more resistance.

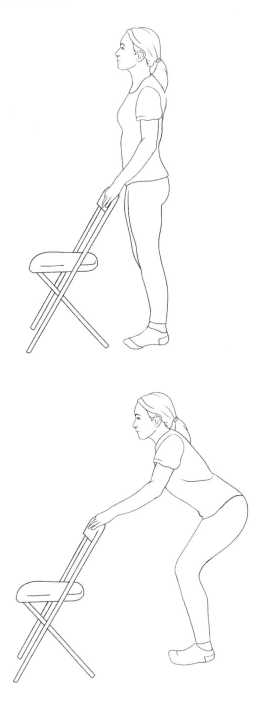

Hip Extension

1. Stand up holding a chair or wall to balance yourself.

2. Gently swing your leg behind you. Make sure to keep your knee straight.

3. Return back to the ground. Repeat on each leg for 10 reps each.

* Inhale while pressing the leg back, exhale while bringing it back. Keep your body upright and tighten your stomach muscles. Add an ankle weight to make it harder.

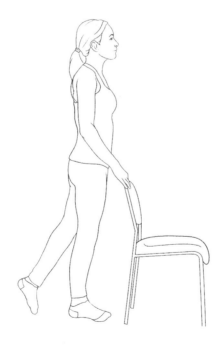

Never forget how important static stretching is! Here are some static stretches to try.

Quad Stretch

1. Stand tall with your hand on a stability tool, such as the wall, a counter, or a chair.

2. Bend your knee and raise your ankle behind you and bring it up towards your hand.

3. Reach around your foot and grab your ankle from the outside.

4. Pull your ankle towards your back.

5. Stand up straight. You should feel a pull in the front of your thigh. Hold for 20 seconds.

6. Return to rest then repeat on the other side.

*This stretch may be difficult for some, which is fine! Simply pick the best stretches for you.

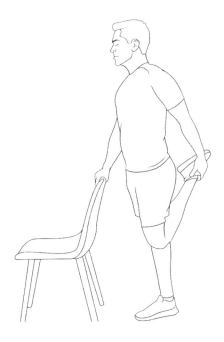

Inner Thigh Stretch

1. Stand with your feet wider apart than your shoulders. Have a chair in front of you for stability and support.

2. Bend your right leg and lean to the right, while keeping the left leg straight. Point your right foot toes out to 45 degrees and keep your left toes pointed ahead. You should feel a pull on the inside of your left thigh. Breathe normally, in the nose and out the mouth.

3. Hold this for 20 – 30 seconds, then switch sides.

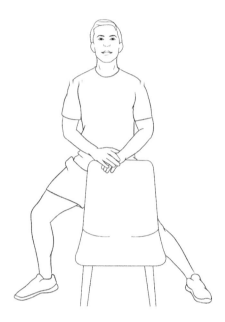

Chair Hamstring Stretch

1. Sit in a chair and scoot to the edge of the seat. Breathe normally.

2. Extend your leg out in front of you and keep your toes pointed to the ceiling. Make sure your upper body and torso are facing your legs.

3. Keep your back straight and lean forward. You'll feel the stretch in the back of your thigh.

4. Hold for 20 – 30 seconds and repeat on the other side.

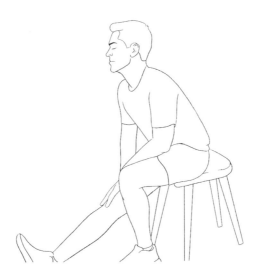

Seated Hip Stretch

1. Sit comfortably in a chair. Breathe normally.

2. Raise your knee to your chest and interlace your fingers across the front of your shin.

3. Pull your knee in and hug it for 20 – 30 seconds.

4. Return your leg back to the ground for rest.

* To make the stretch deeper, pull the knee towards the opposite shoulder.

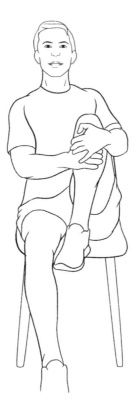

Lower body exercise can help with arthritis. Though you can't reverse the effects completely, doing these exercises daily can certainly help you with increased functional motion. You'll see that your ability to do certain things around the house, like reaching for that jar on top shelf or tying your shoes, has become significantly easier. The next set of exercises work your abdominal and hip flexor muscles together and will help with your back aches.

8

OH, IT'S MY BACK!

Imagine this-

You have a bookshelf full of amazing books that you've collected over the years. You're bored of the way they are arranged. You want to bring more categorization to your bookshelf. So one fine day, you set to rearrange the bookshelf. You take down your books one by one and sit down on the floor reminiscing about the time you bought each one of those books and where and how you read it. You come across some books that you know you've read, but you can't quite remember the names of all its characters, for some recalling even the protagonists' name is hard. You softly smile to yourself cherishing sweet memories and pile up books upon books, one pile has all the classics, the other has all your piano books from back when you learned to play your piano, yet another pile has your gardening books, another has your collection of myriad self-help books and so on. You get up and try to pick up 7-8 books from one pile for the ease of carrying them back to your bookshelf. Not only do you find it hard to stand up after having sat down cross-legged on the floor for so long, but also your back can't take the strain of picking up a pile of 7-8 books at once.

Do you think this could be you in the story? If yes, the following back exercises are definitely going to help you rearrange that bookshelf much more smoothly.

Warming up is part of the workout! Check out some of the warmup exercises in the previous chapters. Your back is in control of all of your movement. Stretching and strengthening the back can lead to many full- body benefits. Let's talk about some stretching exercises for your back!

Lying Knees to Chest

1. Lay on your back on the ground or another flat surface with your knees bent.

2. Bring both of your knees to your chest and hug them.

3. Hold them against you for 15 seconds. Breathe in as you raise your legs up. Exhale as you lower your feet.

4. Return your feet back to the ground.

5. Repeat for a total of 10 reps.

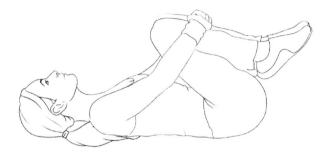

Supine Twist Stretch

1. Lay on your back on the ground or another flat surface with your knees bent. Place your hands behind your head or stretched out beside you.

2. Twist your hips to the right and let your knees fall over to the floor, as low as comfortable. Try to keep your upper back on the ground. It's okay if it lifts a little or your knees don't touch the ground. Hold for 15 seconds.

3. Return your knees to their position in the middle.

4. Repeat on both sides for a total of 10 reps each.

* Breathe normally, in through the nose and out through the mouth.

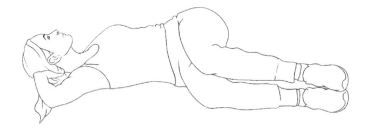

Prone Bridge Stretch

1. Lay on your stomach on the ground or other flat surface.

2. Prop yourself up on your elbows, extending your back.

3. Straighten out your arms until you're holding yourself up.

4. You should feel a gentle stretch in your back. Don't over-stretch and if there's pain then stop.

5. Lower yourself down to the starting position. Repeat 3 – 5 times.

* Breathe normally, in through the nose and out through the mouth.

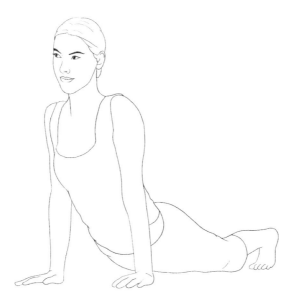

Pelvic Tilt Stretch

1. Lay on your back on the ground or another flat surface with your knees bent.

2. Tighten your abs and push your lower back into the ground. (Imagine trying to pull your belly button down towards the ground.

3. Hold for a count of 10 then return to normal. Breathe normally, through your nose and out of your mouth.

4. Repeat for a total of 10 times.

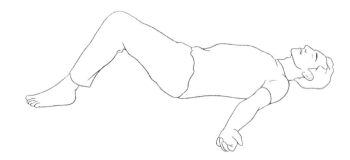

Bridging Stretch

1. Lay on your back on the ground or another flat surface with your knees bent.

2. Push your feet into the floor and raise your hips and butt off of the ground.

3. Hold for 10 seconds, then return to the starting position. Breathe normally.

4. Repeat 3 – 5 times.

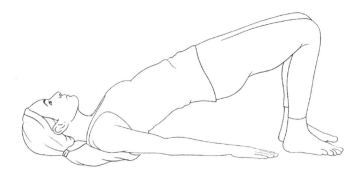

Cat-Cow Stretch

1. Kneel on the floor or other hard surface on your hands and knees.

2. Arch your back up towards the ceiling like an upset cat. Breathe in through the nose and out through the mouth.

3. Hold for 5 seconds.

4. Return to normal.

5. Lower your stomach to the ground. Press your belly button towards the floor as best as you can.

6. Return to normal then repeat for 3 – 5 rounds.

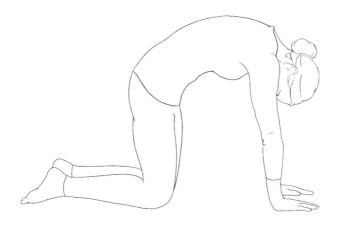

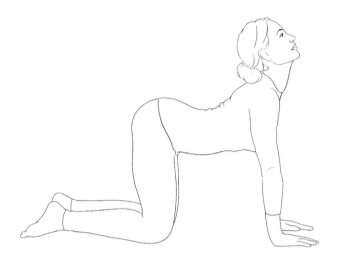

Seated Forward Curl Stretch

1. Sit in a chair with your feet on the ground. Take a deep breath.

2. Exhale as you curl your neck and upper and lower back forward until your chest is on your thighs. You should also be able to touch the ground. Breathe normally.

3. Hold for 10 seconds, then sit up straight. Inhale as you raise to the beginning position.

4. Repeat 3 – 5 times.

* Keep movements slow and smooth. Don't fling down and fly back into your chair. This can make you dizzy or nauseous.

If you experience dizziness, pain, or nausea then stop the stretch.

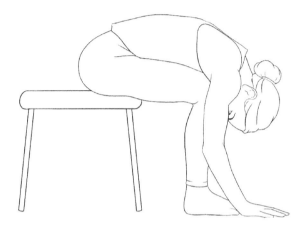

Side Stretch

1. Place your palms flat on the outer sides of your thighs. Bend your trunk to the left, letting your hand slide down your thigh as far as you can, safely.

2. Raise your right hand up over your head and reach to the left.

2. Hold for 10 seconds, then raise back to the beginning.

3. Repeat on both sides for 10 reps each.

* Breathe normally. Do not over-bend. If you feel pain or dizziness, stop the stretch. Have something or someone near you in case you lose balance.

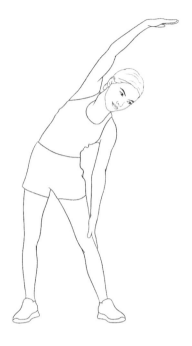

Back Strength Exercises

Bent Knee Raise

1. Lay on your back on the ground or another flat surface with your knees bent.

2. Tighten the abdominals. Think of sinking your belly button down.

3. Raise your knees, one at a time, up to your chest.

4. Hold for 5 seconds, then return your feet flat to the ground.

* Inhale while bringing the knees up, exhale while lowering them. To make it harder, lower one leg at a time.

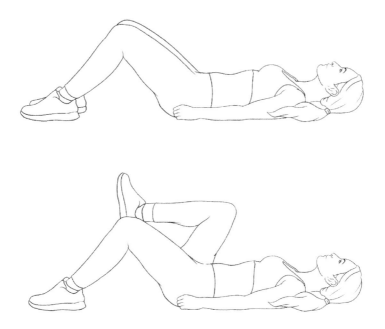

Curl Ups

1. Lay on your back with your knees bent.

2. Cross your arms across your chest and hold each of your shoulders.

3. Breathe in and lift your shoulders off the ground.

4. Pause and hold, keeping your stomach muscles tight.

5. Exhale as you lower back down.

* Breathe in through your nose and out through your mouth. Keep your back flat on the floor. You can put your hands behind your head to avoid neck pain.

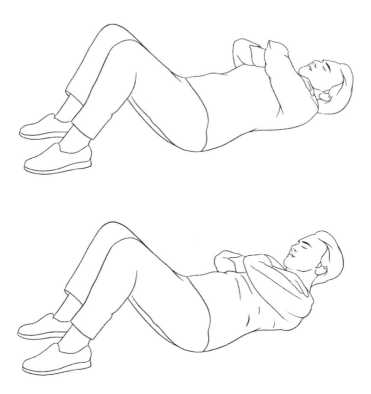

Back Extension

1. Lay face down on the ground with your palms flat against the ground by your face.

2. Push yourself up and prop yourself on your elbows. Use your back muscles as much as you can when you are going up.

3. Return back to the down position.

4. Repeat for 10 reps.

* Inhale while pushing up onto your elbows. Exhale when lowering them down. Keep your hips on the floor.

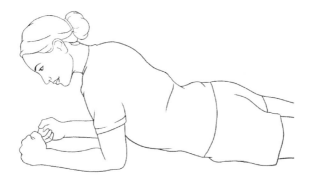

Leg Extension

1. Get on your hands and knees on the ground or other flat surface.

2. Press your right leg straight back. (Think of a horse kicking).

3. Keep your leg parallel with your back.

4. Bring the knee back to the ground and repeat on the other side.

5. Complete 10 reps on each leg.

* Inhale while pressing your leg out and exhaling while bringing it down. Try to keep your hips still. To make it more of a workout, try to raise your foot to the ceiling.

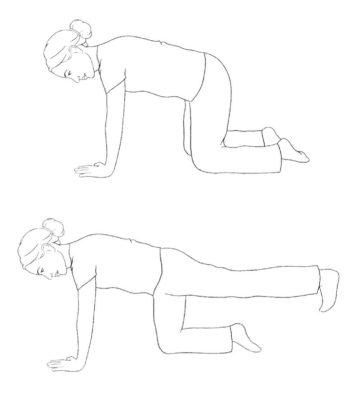

Bridging

1. Lay on your back with your knees bent. Place your hands at your sides or under your bottom.

2. Push your bottom off the floor, leaving only your feet, shoulders, arms, and head on the ground.

3. Repeat for 10 reps.

* Keep your stomach muscles tight and your back straight. Breathe as you press up and exhale as you lower. Hug your legs after the exercise to help relax the muscles. To make it

tougher, hold one leg straight while using the other to push the body up.

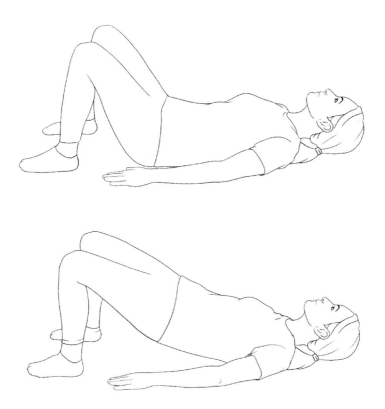

Pelvic Tilt

1. Lay on your back with your knees bent.

2. Tighten your stomach muscles and press your lower back into the floor.

3. Repeat for 10 reps.

* Exhale while tilting back and inhale while returning to the beginning. You can put your hands behind your hips. To increase strength, press your spine into the floor and raise your arms.

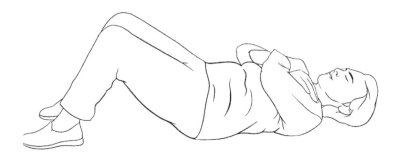

Sit Backs

1. Sit on your bottom with your knees bent and feet out in front of you.

2. Cross your arms across your chest and lean back as far as you can, without letting your feet leave the ground, and pause.

3. Return to the sitting position.

4. Repeat for 10 reps.

* Tighten your abdominals. If your feet start to come off of the floor, sit up. Keep your back as straight as possible. To increase the burn, hold a weight in each hand and extend one leg out as you lean back.

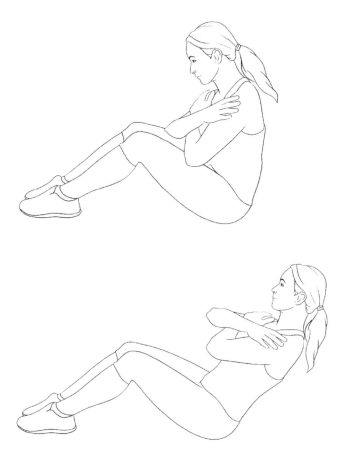

Arm Raises on Back

1. Lay on your back with knees bent. Rest arms by your side.

2. Raise your right arm up to the ceiling, as if you're reaching out to touch it.

3. Return your arm to the ground. Repeat on both sides for 10 reps each.

* Inhale as your raise, exhale as you lower. Keep your spine straight and don't twist or rotate. Don't swing the arm up and down. To make it tougher, add a weight to your hand and extend the opposite leg at the same time.

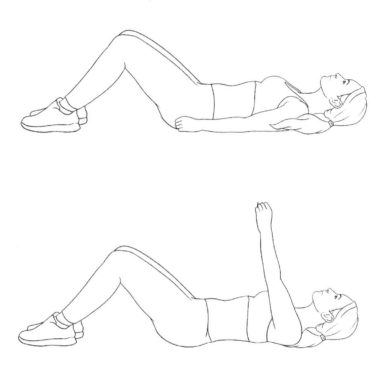

Arm Raises on Knees

1. Get onto all-fours, on your hands and knees on the floor.

2. Stretch your arm out in front of you, raising it until it's even with your eyesight.

3. Hold this, then lower back to the ground.

4. Repeat for 10 reps on each arm.

* Inhale while bringing the arm up, exhale while lowering it down. Keep your hands and knees shoulder-width apart. You can also do this exercise in bed. To increase intensity, add a weight or extend the opposite leg at the same time.

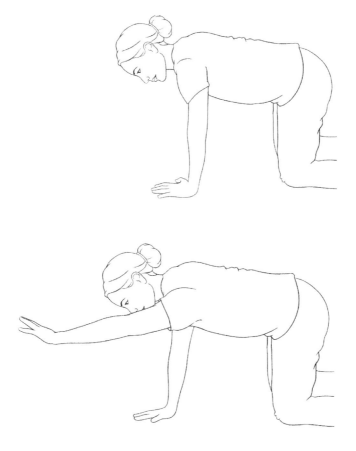

Hip Flexion

1. Get onto your hands and knees.

2. Press back, letting your butt lower towards your feet.

3. Leave your hands in place and keep your back as straight as you can.

4. Return to the beginning motion. Repeat for 10 reps.

* Breathe out as you're moving back and breathe in as you're returning to the beginning phase. To make it harder, pause after you push back for 10 seconds or double the reps.

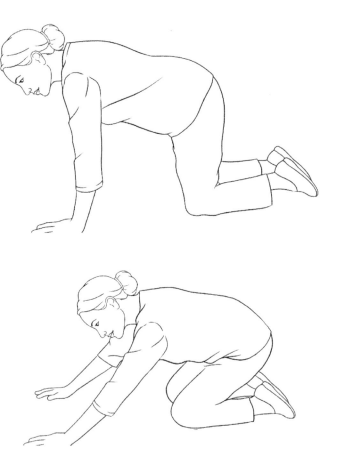

Reverse Straight Leg Raise

1. Lay on your back and tighten your stomach muscles.

2. Bring your right knee toward your chest. Keep your left leg straight.

3. Straighten your leg and lower it back down.

4. Repeat for 10 reps on each leg.

* Inhale while pulling the knee up, exhaling while lowering it down. Holder for longer or add an ankle weight to make it tougher.

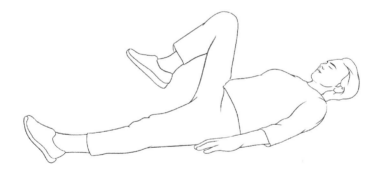

Static Stretching

Stretching is an essential part to healthy exercise. Stretching helps improve recovery, reduce DOMS, and cool muscles down. Try out these back stretches after your back training exercises.

Neck and Chest Stretch

1. Sit with your feet on the floor.

2. Interlace your fingers on the back of your neck.

3. Lean left, tilting your elbow down.

4. Raise up, then lean right.

5. Repeat for 10 reps on each side.

* Breathe in through your nose and out through your mouth. Keep your butt flat on the chair and try to only move your upper body.

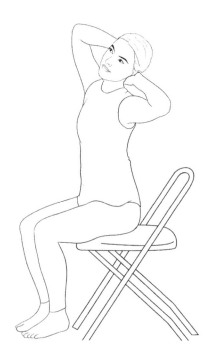

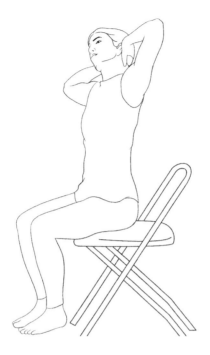

Seated Gentle Backbend

1. Sit with your feet on the floor.

2. Push your hands into your lower back and inhale.

3. Exhale and arch your back, leading with the head. Keep your head and chin lifted up.

4. Hold this position for 5 deep breaths.

5. Slowly and gently return to normal. Repeat 3 – 5 times.

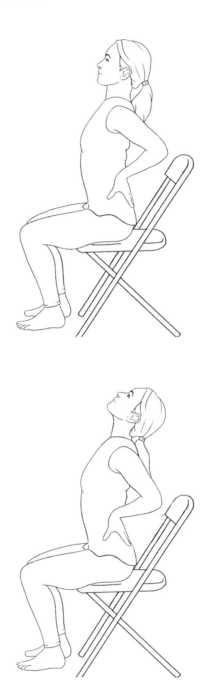

Reach Back

1. Sit with your back straight and your feet on the ground.

2. Take a deep breath and exhale, reaching behind you and interlacing your fingers. If you cannot interlace your fingers, simply grab either wrist or elbow.

3. Inhale and feel your spine grow longer as you sit up.

4. Roll shoulders up and back, moving the shoulder blades.

5. Gently straighten your arms or pull your hands in opposite directions.

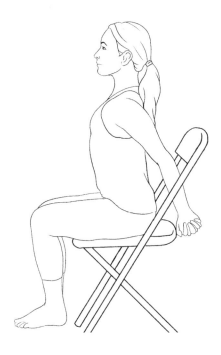

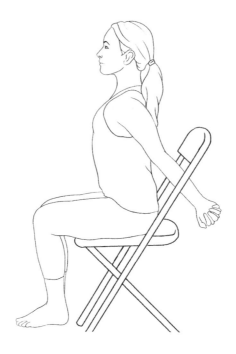

Seated Cat-Cow

1. Sitting down with your feet on the ground, place your palms on your knees with your fingers facing inwards towards each other.

2. Inhale. As you exhale, press into your hands, and arch your back. Your face should be to the sky, and you'll feel like you're poking your butt out.

3. Inhale and bring the chest in, rounding the back and curving it towards the ceiling.

4. Repeat this exercise, slowly, 3 – 5 times.

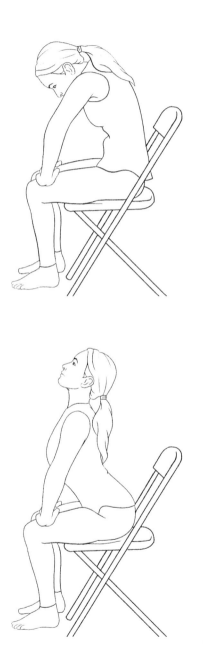

Gentle Twist

1. Sit with your back straight and your feet on the ground.

2. Edge towards the seat but make sure you're stable.

3. Inhale and lift your arms over your head. Think of your spine lengthening.

4. Turn to the right and place your left hand on the outside of your right knee.

5. Place the other hand wherever is comfortable and hold yourself in this twist.

6. Take 3 – 5 deep breaths before releasing. Perform at least 2 stretches on either side.

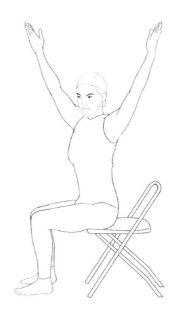

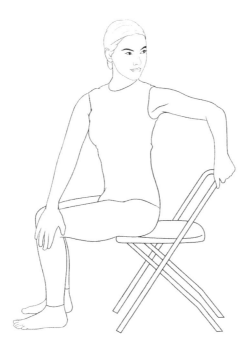

Static stretching should be comfortable and relaxing. This is going to help get you better situated for your next workout. Doing these exercises with consistency will help you with all your back issues. Joint pain, backache, and the feeling of tiredness raining all over your everyday parade are not highly uncommon as you age. But if you work out regularly, it gets easier. Having your mobility, flexibility, balance, and strength back can make getting older with every passing year, not so bad. What do you know, if you continue with these workouts, it might even be awesome!

9

THE CORE OF TRAINING

Benny had been having some back pain for a couple of weeks. He assured his wife and family he was fine and refused to go to the doctor. Benny was afraid of what the doctor might say. He was having trouble sleeping and taking over the counter reliever to put off some of the pain. After some time, Benny noticed he was having more trouble than normal when leaning over to pick something up. Finally, Benny's wife made him go to a doctor. After thorough tests and checkups, the doctor said that Benny just had a weak core.

Your abdominals, back, hip, and pelvis muscles, along with the muscles along your spine, together make up your core. A strong core prevents you from fall risks, poor balance, and limited mobility. To be honest, every movement your body makes is more or less generated from your core, which is why it is called…well… the core. If you have a weak core, all other muscles have to work that much harder to contribute to your movement. This can result in serious injuries as you age which makes core workout all the more important for older adults.

WHAT IS THE CORE?

The core is made up of all the muscles in the trunk. Every time you twist, turn, step, or move, you're using your core. Some of the main muscles in the core include:

- Glutes. The gluteus maximus is the thick, meaty muscle in your butt. They help you stand up, push yourself upstairs, and walk around the grocery store. The gluteus medius is a smaller muscle on both sides of your bottom. They are responsible for keeping you steady when you move.
- Rectus abdominis. The rectus abdominis is the 6-pack you see on the stomach. This muscle extends from the rib cage to pubic bone. This muscle flexes and bends the trunk.
- Obliques. Obliques consist of external oblique muscles on each side of the trunk. Internal muscles are also included below the external obliques. These muscles are responsible for moving your trunk side to side.
- Transverse abdominis. This muscle is the deepest abdominal muscle and works to stabilize the pelvis

and low back. It helps you breathe as well.

- <u>Multifidus and Erector Spinae</u>. These muscles bend and straighten the spine.
- <u>Psoas</u>. This muscle connects the legs to the trunk and helps bend the hips.

Exercising these core muscles are great for many reasons. Strong core muscles:

- Improve posture and reduce back pain.
- Help with daily activities and movements.
- Improves coordination and balance.
- Support the spine.

Working out the core is a great way to stay healthy and proactive as a senior. Never forget, however, to warm up. You can do a couple of these warm-up exercises to get ready to exercise your core.

Spine Warmup #1

1. Sit in a chair with your spine straight.

2. Have your legs extended out from the chair but keep your feet flat on the ground.

3. Place the palms of your hands on your lap.

4. Lean forward, running your hands down your legs as far as you can without causing pain.

5. Lean back running your hands back up your legs until you are sitting straight up again with your hands in your lap

6. Repeat 5 times breathing normally throughout the exercise

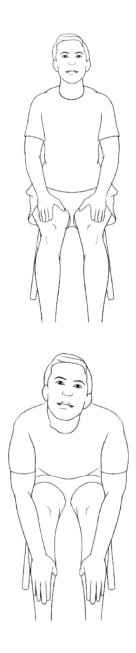

Spine warmup #2

1. Sit down in a chair with your spine straight.

2.Place your right hand on your left shoulder and your left hand on your right shoulder making an X across your chest with your arms

3.Lean forward and touch your elbows to your knees

4.Lean back until you are sitting straight again

5.Repeat 5 times breathing normally throughout the exercise

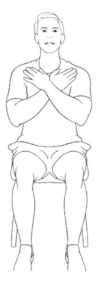

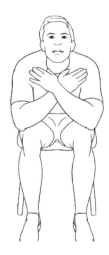

Core Exercises

Good Mornings

1. Sit comfortably in a chair. Sit up and try to pull your belly button back towards your spine.

2. Bend your elbows at 90 degrees, then hold your arms on either side of you up, with your palms facing out. (Think of being told to freeze and put your hands up.)

3. Stretched your elbows back to open your chest.

4. Keep the back straight and lean forward down to the knees.

5. Pause for a second then return to the sitting position. Repeat for 5 – 10 reps.

* Breathe out as you lean down, breathe in as you raise up. Add weights to improve intensity.

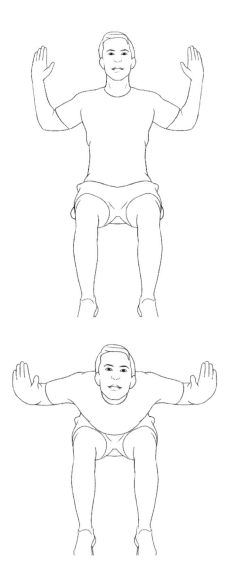

Leg Lifts

1. Sit up in your chair and hold onto the sides for leverage.

2. Raise your right knee into the air.

3. Focus on using your stomach to lift your knee.

4. Lower your leg back to the ground.

5. Repeat for 10 reps on each side.

* Breathe in as you lift your leg. Breathe out as you lower it. Use ankle weights or increase reps to increase difficulty.

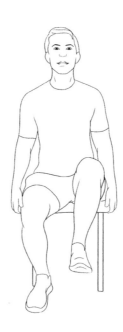

Heel and Toe Taps

1. Sit upright in your chair and hold the sides for support.

2. Focus on pulling your belly button in towards your spine.

3. Stretch both legs out in front of you and rest your heels on the ground. Your toes should be pointing up.

4. Bend your legs up and tuck your feet under the chair with only your toes on the ground.

5. Return to pressing your heels out. Repeat for 5 – 10 reps.

* If you have knee pain, do not bend them as deep when doing the toe taps. Breathe out as you're pushing your heels out. Breathe in as you are bringing your toes underneath. Increase reps or add ankle weights to improve outcomes.

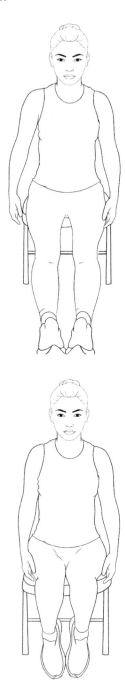

Seated Side Bends

1. Sit in the chair with your feet flat on the floor.

2. Put one hand behind your head. Take the other and reach, beside you, towards the floor.

3. Lean over like you're going to touch the floor.

4. Raise back up, focusing on squeezing your side.

5. Repeat 8 – 10 times on both sides.

* Breathe in as you raise up. Breathe out as you raise down. Try not to lean forward. Tilt only as far as you're comfortable. Stop if you experience pain or dizziness. Hold your home-made water bottle to make it more difficult.

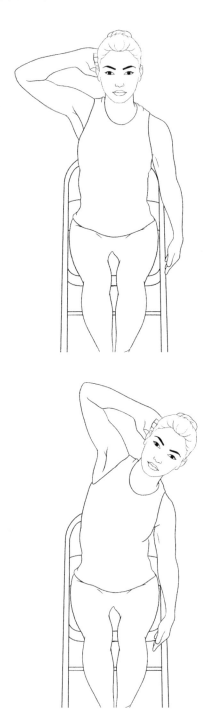

The Bridge

1. Lay flat on your back and bend your knees. Keep your feet on the floor.

2. Squeeze your stomach muscles and lift your hips to make a straight line between your chest and knees. Hold for 3 seconds.

3. Keep your back in a straight line, as well.

4. Return to resting position. Repeat for 10 reps.

* Breathe out as you raise up, breathe in as you lower down. Hold for 5 seconds or increase reps for increased intensity.

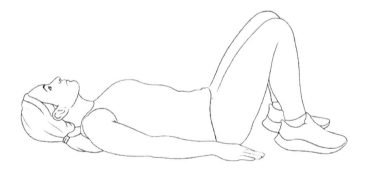

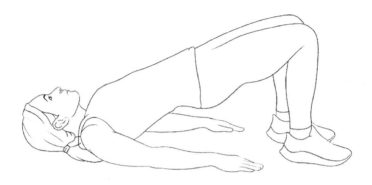

The Superman

1. Lay face down on a flat surface.

2. Stretch your arms out in front of you. (Like you're Superman flying!)

3. Raise your head.

4. Rise your right arm and left leg about 2 inches off the ground.

5. Lower them. Raise your left arm and your right leg. Lower them.

6. Repeat for 10 reps on each side.

* Breathe in as you're raising your limbs. Breathe out as you're lowering them down. Add ankle or wrist weights to make this more challenging. If you feel back pain, stop the exercise.

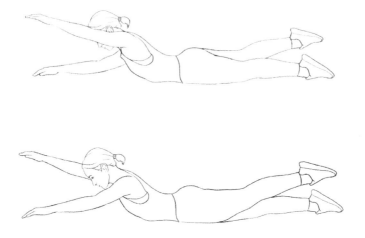

Seated Forward Roll-Ups

1. Sit up tall with your bottom near the front edge of the chair.

2. Stretch your legs and arms out in front of you.

3. Roll your shoulders forward and lower your trunk, arching your back as your lower and reach for your toes.

4. Slowly roll back up, arching the back and rolling the shoulders back.

5. Return to sitting position. Complete 5 – 10 reps.

* If you feel pain or dizziness, stop the exercise. Focus on using your stomach muscles to lower yourself and bring yourself back up. Breathe in as you roll up and out as you roll down. Hold your crafty weights to make it more challenging.

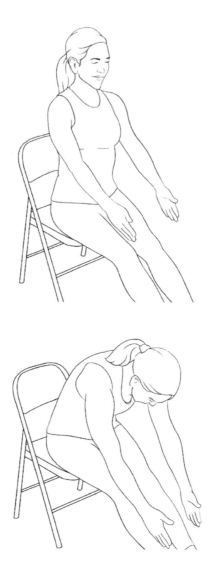

Seated Half Rollbacks

1. Sit comfortably towards the front edge of the seat.

2. Bend your knees at a 90-degree angle and keep your feet flat on the floor.

3. Lift your arms in front of you to make a circle. (You might look like a basketball hoop).

4. Round your back and focus on scooping in your abdominals inward, like you're pulling them to your back.

5. Use your abs to slowly return to the starting position. Repeat for 10 reps.

* Breathe in as you lower down, breathe out as you raise up.

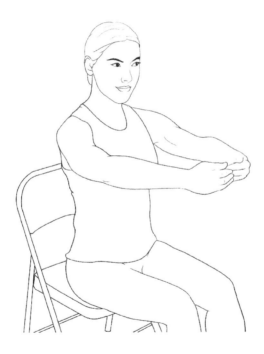

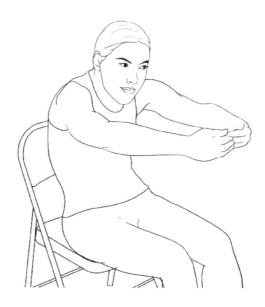

Forearm Planks

1. Lay face down on the floor with your forearms on the ground. Make sure your elbows are under your shoulders.

2. Squeeze your core and press down with your forearms, raising your butt and body off of the ground.

3. Your body should be in a straight slant from head to toe.

4. Pull your belly button to your spine.

5. Squeeze your hips and glutes to keep them from dipping towards the floor.

6. Hold for 30 seconds or as long as you can, without going over 1 minute.

* Breathe normally, in through your nose and out through your mouth. This may be one of the more challenging moves of the chapter. You can rest your knees on the ground or check out the alternate movement below.

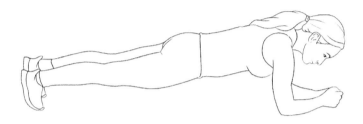

Full-Body Rollups

1. Lay flat on your back on a flat surface.

2. Raise your hands up and out in front of you.

3. Use your abs to squeeze and pull you up. Try to keep your feet on the ground.

4. Slowly roll up and forward, reaching to touch your toes.

5. Slowly roll back and onto the ground, using your abs to keep you steady.

6. Repeat for 5 – 10 reps.

* Breathe normally, in through the nose and out through the mouth. If you feel pain or dizziness, stop the movements.

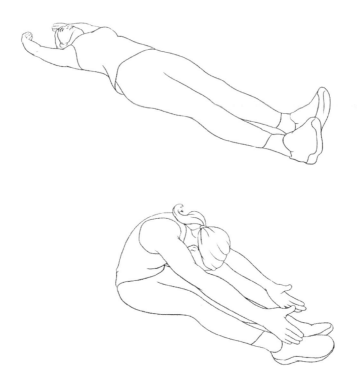

Static Stretching

Repeat static stretches from the end of chapter 8.

Benny began a 4-month exercise program that he created with his doctor. After a few days he noticed an improvement in pain. After a few weeks he noticed he was able to pick stuff up easier than before. At the end of his 4-month plan, Benny was stronger and healthier than he was before. His back pain had gone down significantly and he was no longer having trouble sleeping.

Seniors are one of the groups who should be doing core strengthening exercises regularly because of the benefits they yield. Not only is core strengthening beneficial for posture and back pain, but it also improves balance. Having strong balance is especially important for seniors. In the next chapter, we will see some easy yet super effective balance training exercises.

10

BALANCE TRAINING EXERCISES

As we grow older, our balance fades away. This is due to changes in our hearing and ear structures, any medications we may be taking, or medical conditions we're experiencing. Ordinarily we take our balance for granted but have you ever lost your footing while going down a flight of stairs or on icy pavement because it is too slippery? Do you remember flailing your arms like your life depended on it to find your footing? Do you remember the thump…thump…thump…of your accelerated heartbeats in your ears? Do you remember how your balance saved you in those times?

As you get older, your balance declines naturally and you become susceptible to fall risks. But this can be managed and minimized by regular balance training. Read on to find some simple home exercises that you can add to your weekly workout schedule to improve your balance.

WHY DO SENIORS FALL?

Seniors are one of the most at-risk groups for falls that can lead to injury. This is because of:

Decreases and changes in sight, making it harder to see clearly.

- Weaker muscles in the hips and legs, making it more difficult to walk.
- Spinal degeneration or other conditions may make it hard to stand up tall.
- Many medications that can cause disorientation or dizziness.
- Longer reaction times if something trips us or gets in our way.
- Lightheadedness due to conditions such as blood pressure and diabetes.

HOW DOES OUR BALANCE WORK, REALLY?

When we get on the elevator, walk across the grass, or trip over an object, we depend on our balance to keep us upright. Our bodies use a number of aspects to improve and control balance. Without these tools, the body may have a harder time keeping up with our balance needs. Our balance comes from information from our eyes, vestibular system, and joints.

Visual cues tell us about our environments. They help us prepare for barriers and obstacles that could lead to trips and falls. The vestibular system is in our ears. There is a canal filled with fluid inside our ears that gives us information on where our head is in relation to space and gravity. Feedback from joints also helps our muscles decide which direction we may be moving and improves reaction time. When our visual and vestibular information is damaged or not operating at its best, it can lead to dizziness.

If you're experiencing moderate to severe balance or dizziness issues, check with your doctor to rule out certain conditions or events that may be causing this, such as vertigo, ear infections, Meniere's disease, or drug interactions.

WARMING UP

Regardless of the activity you're performing, it's always important to complete your warm-up. Try some of these exercises before your next balance training session.

Neck Stretches

1. Stand tall near a chair. You can use this for balance if you need it.

2. Look to the right and hold for 5 seconds.

3. Look to the left and hold for 5 seconds.

4. Look at the ceiling for 5 seconds.

5. Tuck the chin and look down for 5 seconds.

6. Repeat 2 3 times.

* Breathe normally, in through the nose and out through the mouth. Dizziness may occur. Hold your chair and breathe. If the dizziness doesn't go away, do not continue with the stretch.

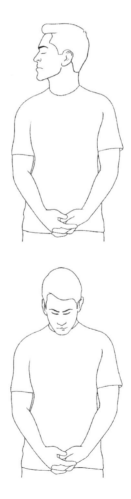

Shoulder Stretch

1. Stand comfortably with your hands at your side and your thumbs facing out.

2. Slowly reach your arms out and up high above your head keeping your arms straight.

3. Hold your arms in the up position for 3 seconds feeling the stretch in your shoulders.

4. Slowly lower them down. Repeat 10 times.

* Breathe normally. Keep slow, controlled movements.

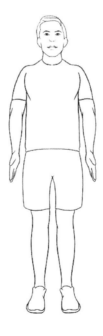

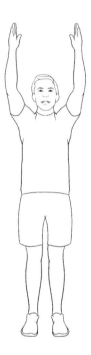

Shoulder Rotations

1. Stand tall.

2. Raise your shoulders to your ears then roll them in a circle behind you. Repeat 10 times. Try to roll them as wide as you can.

3. Roll your shoulders in front of you 10 times.

4. Return to resting position. Repeat 2 – 3 times.

* Breathe normally, in through the nose and out through the mouth. If there's pain, stop the exercise, or don't roll your shoulders as wide.

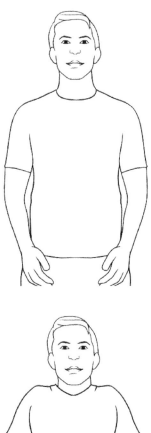

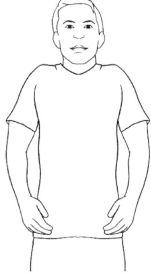

Hip Flexions

1. Stand near a wall or other form of support.

2. Gently raise one leg until your knee is in a straight line with your hip.

3. Pause then lower onto the ground.

4. Repeat on each leg for 10 reps.

* Focus on using your hips to raise your knee. Go slow and use support when needed. Breathe normally.

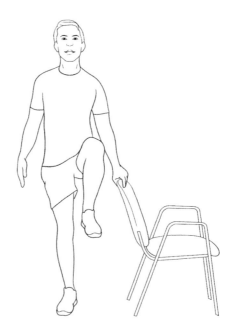

Elbow Movements

1. Stand with your arms at your side.

2. Turn your palms towards you as you reach up and touch your shoulders.

3. Return your hand to your side.

4. Repeat for 10 reps.

* Breathe in as you raise your arms and out as you lower them.

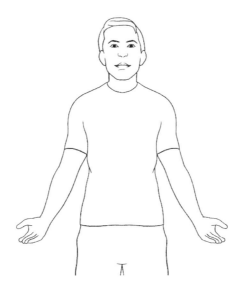

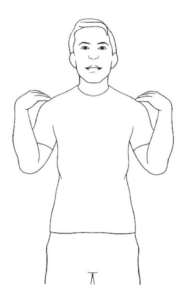

Balance Training Exercises

Balance training exercises should be completed standing up to be most effective. Always have another object, wall, or person nearby in case you lose your balance. Check with your doctor before completing any balance exercises. You can make balancing exercises difficult by adding ankle or wrist weights, or removing your hands from any support device (or only use a few fingers to hold on).

Single Limb Stance

1. Stand with your arms at your side and legs and feet together. Have a wall or chair around for support.

2. Lift one foot about 6 – 7 inches off the ground.

3. Hold for 10 seconds, then return the foot to the ground.

4. Repeat on the other leg.

* Breathe in through the nose and out through the mouth. If you find you're having trouble, try only lifting it off the ground an inch or two and if you feel like you're going to fall, simply lower your foot and try again.

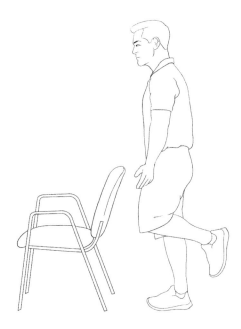

Eye Tracking

1. Stand comfortable.

2. Hold your thumb about 18 inches from your face. Keep your elbow bent.

3. Move your thumb to the right and follow it with your eyes, as far right as you can.

4. Move your thumb to the left and follow it with your eyes, as far left as you can.

5. Return to center. Repeat 2 – 3 times.

* Breathe normally. Try not to use your head, only your eyes.

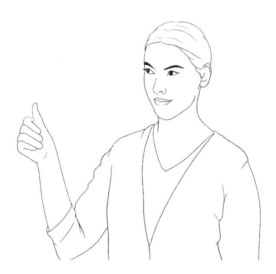

1. Stand comfortably.

2. Hold your thumb about 18 inches from your face. Keep your elbow bent.

3. Move your thumb up and follow it with your eyes, as far right as you can.

4. Move your thumb down and follow it with your eyes, as far down as you can.

5. Return to center. Repeat 2 – 3 times.

* Breathe normally. Try not to use your head, only your eyes.

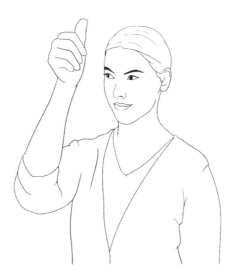

1. Stand comfortable.

2. Hold your thumb at arms length straight in front of you.

3. Moving your thumb to the right as far as you can. This time move your head as you keep your eyes on your thumb.

4. Move your thumb to the right as far as you can moving your head as your eyes stay focused on your thumb.

5. Move back to center and repeat 2- 3 times

---

1. Hold your thumb at arms length straight in front of you.

2. Move your thumb up as far as you can moving your head as you stay focused on you thumb.

3. Be careful not to lose your balance. Stand near something stable that you can grab just in case you need to steady yourself.

4. Move your thumb down as far as you can.

5. Return to center

6. Repeat 2- 3 times.

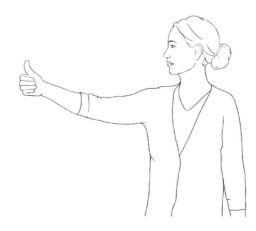

Clock Reach

1. Stand near a counter or chair and hold for support.

2. Imagine you are standing on a clock and 12 o'clock is in front of you and 6 o'clock is behind you.

3. Lift your right leg and point your arm to 12 (right in front of you). Move your right arm to 3 o'clock (out to your side) then to 6 o'clock (straight behind you).

4. Repeat 3 – 5 times on each side.

* Breathe normally, in through the nose and out through the mouth. If reaching towards 6 is painful, just reach as far as you can.

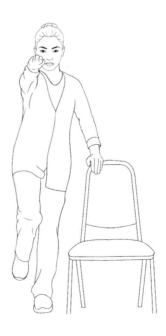

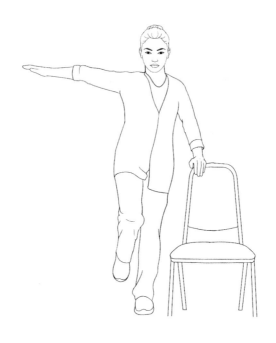

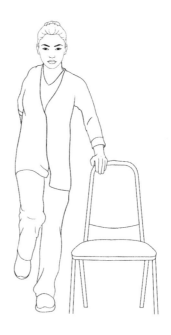

Staggered Stance

1. Stand with your arms at your side and legs and feet together. Have a wall or chair around for support.

2. Put your right heel in front of your left toe. Hold this for 10 seconds, then repeat on the other side.

3. Repeat 3 – 5 times.

* Breathe normally, in through the nose and out through the mouth. You can keep your arms out to the side to help with balance. Practice on the floor with tape to be more accurate.

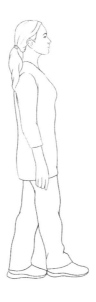

Single Limb Stance with Arm

1. Hold onto a chair and stand with your feet together.

2. Raise your right hand into the air.

3. Raise your right leg off of the floor. Hold this position for 10 seconds, then relax to the floor.

4. Repeat on the other side. Repeat 3 – 5 times.

* Breathe normally, in through the nose and out through the mouth.

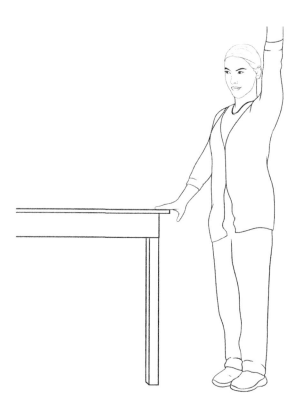

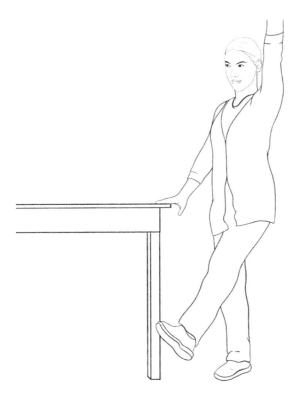

Balancing Wand

1. Find a long, thin, wand-like object. (You can sometimes unscrew the head of a broom and use the broomstick).

2. Hold it in your dominant hand straight up. Keep your palm flat and balance the object on your hand, on its end.

3. Balance as long as you can.

* Be cautious not to hit yourself in the face if it falls. Ensure there's no one around you or anything breakable. Sit up tall and keep your elbow bent.

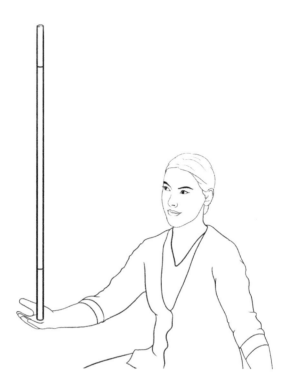

Knee Marching

1. Stand by a wall or chair with your legs shoulder width apart.

2. Raise one knee as high as you can, comfortably.

3. Lower, then raise the other leg.

4. Repeat for 10 times on each leg.

* Breathe normally, inhale through the nose and exhale through the mouth. Keep your chest up and looking ahead.

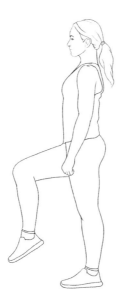

Body Circles

1. Stand with your feet shoulder width apart and arms at your side.

2. Keep your body straight.

3. Slowly sway around in a circle, leaning forward, then around in a circle.

4. Continue swaying for one minute.

* Have something near in case you lose balance. Try to use legs, feet, toes, and core to keep yourself from falling. Don't hold your breath. Bring your feet together to make it more challenging.

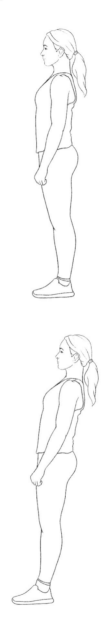

Heel to Toe

1. Start by standing with your feet together, heel to toe.

2. Walk with each foot stepping forward heel to toe. Place the heel of one foot in front of the toe of the other.

3. Walk about 10 steps.

* Wear smooth shoes. Breathe normally, in through the nose and out through the mouth. Lift your chest and look ahead when doing this if you can.

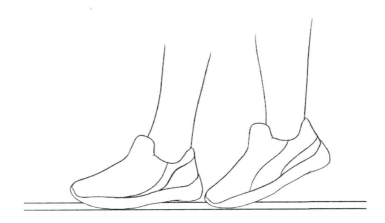

Grapevine

1. Stand with your arms at your sides and your feet together. Step across.

2. You will move your right foot in front of your left foot, crossing it, and resting your right foot on the ground on the opposite side of the left foot.

3. Uncross the left leg, then step across, again, with the right.

4. Walk about 6 – 10 steps, then repeat with the other side.

* Breathe normally, in through the nose and out through the mouth. Wear smooth shoes. Hold onto a chair or other form of support if needed. Use tape for accuracy and try to look ahead if you can.

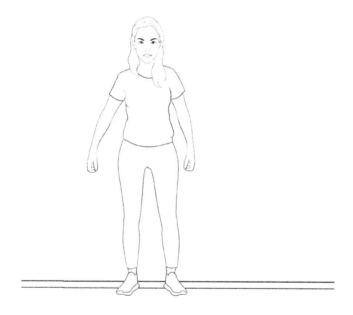

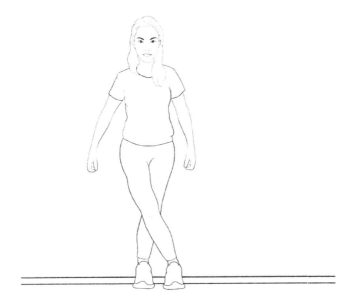

Stepping

1. Find 2 – 3 soft objects and place them on the floor about 12 – 16 inches apart. They could be stuffed animals or pet toys, pillows, slippers, etc.

2. Lift your foot at least 6 inches and step over the object, towards the next one. Pause between each object.

3. Turn around and walk back.

* Breathe normally, in through the nose and out through the mouth. Wear smooth shoes. Hold onto a chair or other form of support if needed.

Side Step Over

1. Find 2 – 3 soft objects and place them on the floor about 12 – 16 inches apart. They could be stuffed animals or pet toys, pillows, slippers, etc.

2. Stand sideways and step over each item, one foot at a time.

3. Pause between objects.

4. Step back the opposite way after stepping over all objects.

* Breathe normally, in through the nose and out through the mouth. Wear smooth shoes. Hold someone's hands if you need support.

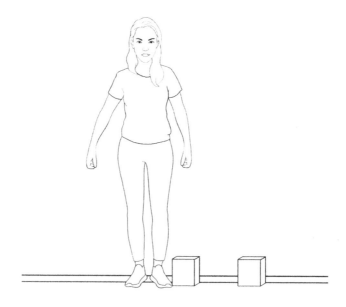

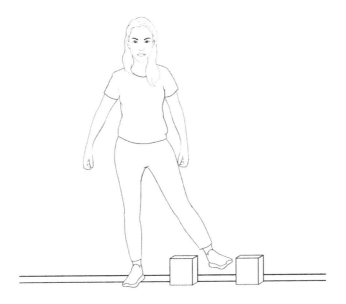

Dynamic Walking

1. Stand in an open and safe room.

2. Slowly walk across the room looking left and right as you step.

3. Repeat 3 – 5 times.

* Breathe normally. Have someone near if you can. Try to walk near a wall in case you lose your balance. You can increase the intensity by reading and turning your head while walking.

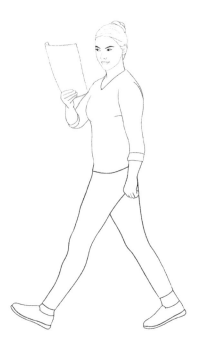

For any kind of workout to be effective what is more important is your consistency. Working out and having an active
lifestyle where you take out at least 40 minutes every day for
your body is guaranteed to make your life much more
fulfilling and the mobility and confidence that you get by
physical fitness are just the tip of the iceberg of benefits that
await you. Happy Training!

CONCLUSION

As we age, our bodies go through a number of changes. We experience:

Slower metabolisms.

- Decreases muscle strength and mass.
- Decreased aerobic capacity.
- Stiff joints.
- Slower reaction times and reflexes.
- Increased bone porosity.
- Fall risks and balance issues.
- Increased body fat.
- Reduced bone density.

Strength and balance training have a number of benefits for the body. Immediate benefits include:

- Decreased pain.
- Boosted energy.
- Improved mood.
- Better mobility.
- Increased and improved circulation.
- Improved quality of life.
- Prevention of social isolation and depression.
- Improved sleep.

Long-term benefits include:

- Increased muscle mass.
- Increased strength.
- Improved muscle tone.
- Stopping certain types of pain.
- Prevent bone fractures.
- Improve and prevent a number of conditions, including diabetes, arthritis, and heart disease.
- Less dependence on others and walking devices.
- Being able to do more of what you want when you want.

As we get older, medical conditions can start to take a toll on our wellbeing. Strength and balance training can improve:

- Heart and lung function
- Blood pressure

- Muscle endurance and strength
- Diabetes
- Brain and thinking
- Inflammation
- Flexibility
- Depression and anxiety

Now that we're at the end of the book, you might be nervous about beginning. Don't worry! There are a number of worries when starting a workout routine. Many people are scared of injuries, expecting a lot of pain, confusion on how to start, dealing with ongoing problems, and worried if they will have enough time. The book covered all you need to know about strength and balance training, as well as how to overcome barriers and prevent new ones!

Let's sum up the most important points of the book.

1. Always check with a doctor before starting any new exercises or programs.

2. Never hold your breath and always rest between exercises and sets.

3. Listen to your body. Exercise should be challenging and uncomfortable, but never painful. If you're experiencing pain, try to ensure you are doing the movement correctly. If the pain doesn't stop, consult your doctor on any underlying conditions or use an alternate exercise.

4. Stay consistent! It can be easy to lose motivation. However, it's about self-discipline! It's about making yourself a priority every day and making the decision to combat the problems that come with aging.

5. If you're exercising alone, it may be beneficial to tell someone you're completing your workouts. This way someone can check in on you afterwards.

6. Don't forget about DOMS (delayed onset muscle soreness). As you continue exercising, DOMS will not be as prevalent as before. If you notice your DOMS is severe after every workout, try decreasing weight, intensity, or reps.

Remember to focus on your posture, breathe right, take proper rest during sets, and increase the intensity of your workout week by week. Don't overdo it. Even if you've never exercised before, you can start now. You'll get to your goal. But not in one day. It is a continuous process and you've rolled your ball. Your job now is to keep it rolling.

Read up and educate yourselves on the correct way of eating the foods you love and still be able to attain your ideal workout goal. There will come a point in your fitness journey where you'll think fitness requires too much effort. But if fitness requires effort, sickness requires a billion times more effort. Fitness is what adds quality to your life.

So, go out there and talk to your friends about this new venture of yours and try to get them on-board too. Having an equally enthusiastic partner makes working out much more fun. But also, remember no two bodies are alike. The restrictions of your body and theirs aren't the same so the progress will look different. Don't compare your workouts and get depressed about the difference in results.

Stay motivated and do these workouts every day. Small victories in the form of agility, ability to do so much more around the house, less painful and stiff joints are not exactly what others can see or measure. But you can feel the change and you know you're improving every day. Put all that you just learned into practice and get started today!

NOTES

American Senior Communities. (2022). The best core exercises for seniors. https://docs.google.com/document/d/ 1YESqWpP6E4kv6MULcs6Q_k_xNq1UeYwKaMsfTIHWLhA/edit

Bain, J. & Chang, L. (25 October 2010). New ideas on proper stretching techniques. *WebMD.* https://www.webmd.com/fitness-exercise/features/new-ideas-on-proper-stretching-techniques

Bedosky, L. (22 April 2022). The best core exercises for seniors. *Get Healthy.* https://gethealthyu.com/best-core-exercises-for-seniors/

Betterhealth. (26 August 2018). Resistance training; Health benefits. https://www.betterhealth.vic.gov.au/health/healthyliving/resistance-training-health-benefits

Blessing, J. (28 December 2018). Importance of warming up. *Wyomissing.* https://www.wyofitness.com/importance-of-warming-up

Borawski, B. (21 June 2011). Coaching tip: The importance of journaling. *Breaking Muscle.* https://breakingmuscle.com/coaching-tip-the-importance-of-journaling/

Brett. (3 February 2016). The ultimate glossary of strength and conditioning terms. *Art of Manliness.* https://www.artofmanliness.com/health-fitness/fitness/the-ultimate-glossary-of-strength-and-conditioning-terms/

Bubnis, D. & Kilroy, D. (15 October 2019). Exercise plan for seniors. *Healthline.* https://www.healthline.com/health/everyday-fitness/senior-workouts

Cavill, N. & Foster, C. (June 2018). Enablers and barriers to older people's participation in strength and balance activities: A review of reviews. *Journal of Frailty, Sarcopenia, & Falls, 3*(2).pp.105-113.doi:10.22540/JFSF-03-105

Cheung, K., Hume, P., and Maxwell, L. (2003). Delayed onset muscle soreness: Treatment strategies and performance factors. *Sports Medicine, 33*(2), pp. 145 - 164. doi: 10.2165/00007256-200333020-00005.

Colberg-Ochs, S. (12 January 2019). Resistance training guidelines for older adults or anyone with reduced mobility. *Diabetes Strong.* https://diabetesstrong.com/resistance-training-guidelines-for-older-adults-or-anyone-with-reduced-mobility/

Culpepper Place. (4 February 2019), The benefits of strength training for senior adults. https://culpepperplaceassistedliving.com/the-benefits-of-strength-training-for-senior-adults/

Dan. (2022). How to study for the HSC. *Pdhpe.net.* https://pdhpe.net/factors-affecting-performance/how-does-training-affect-performance/principles-of-training/specificity/

Eldergym. (2021). 12 best elderly balance exercises for seniors to help prevent falls. https://eldergym.com/elderly-balance/

Eldergym. (2021). Arm workout for seniors and the elderly. https://eldergym.com/arm-workout/

Eldergym. (2021). Benefits of stretching for seniors and the elderly. https://eldergym.com/benefits-of-stretching/

Eldergym. (2021). Chest exercises for seniors and the elderly. https://eldergym.com/chest-exercises/

Eldergym. (2021). Elbow exercises for seniors and the elderly. https://eldergym.com/elbow-exercises/

Eldergym. (2021). Hand exercises for seniors and the elderly. https://eldergym.com/hand-exercises/

Eldergym. (2021). Muscle stretching exercises for seniors and the elderly. https://eldergym.com/muscle-stretching/

Eldergym. (2021). Shoulder rehabilitation exercises for seniors and the elderly. https://eldergym.com/shoulder-rehabilitation-exercises/

Eldergym. (2021). Stretches before exercise. https://eldergym.com/stretches-before-exercise/

Eldergym. (2021). Stretching routines for seniors and the elderly. https://eldergym.com/stretching-routines/

Eldergym Fitness for Seniors. (3 April 2019). Upper body exercises for seniors and the elderly, strength training for seniors. [Video]. *YouTube.* https://www.youtube.com/watch?v=PBMi4Gr_9ls

Fisher, S. (8 April 2021). How to make weights at home 6 different ways. *The Spruce.* https://www.thespruce.com/make-homemade-weights-5115294

Freedom Health Centers. (6 August 2016). Why you need a physical medical exam before starting a new exercise routine. https://freedomhealthcenters.com/why-you-need-a-physical-medical-exam-before-starting-a-new-exercise-routine

Freytag, C. & Blacker, H. (7 October 2021). Basic strength training with good form. *VeryWell Fit.* https://www.verywellfit.com/basic-strength-training-tips-for-good-form-3498161

HUR. (25 October 2017). Why seniors need lower body strength training - for therapists. https://www.hurusa.com/why-seniors-need-lower-body-strength-training-for-therapists/

Invararity, L. & DelCollo, J. (26 October 2021). Stretching exercises for your back. *Very Well Health.* https://www.verywellhealth.com/stretching-exercises-for-your-back-2696357

ISSA. (15 April 2019). The importance of strength training for seniors. https://www.issaonline.com/blog/post/the-importance-of-strength-training-for-seniors

Jackson, H. (19 September 2015). The importance of form over intensity. *Fitness 19.* https://www.fitness19.com/the-importance-of-form-over-intensity/

Johnson, J. & Bubnis, D. (5 January 2021). Which muscle groups can people work out together? *Medical News Today.* https://www.medicalnewstoday.com/articles/muscle-groups-to-work-out-together

Leckie, E. (26 October 2020). How to choose the right exercise footwear for seniors. *Active Beat.* https://www.activebeat.com/fitness/how-to-choose-the-right-exercise-footwear-for-seniors/

Maurice. (2022). Warm up exercises for seniors: Types + why seniors should do them. *Seniors Mobility.* https://seniorsmobility.org/exercises/warm-up-exercises-for-seniors/

Medicareful Living. (19 April 2017). Resting for fitness: The importance of recovery days. https://living.medicareful.com/resting-for-fitness-the-importance-of-recovery-days

More Life Health. (2020). Important legal disclosure. https://morelifehealth.com/disclaimer

More Life Health Seniors. (2 July 2019). Stretching exercises for seniors:

Upper body & lower body stretches for seniors. [Video]. *YouTube*. https://www.youtube.com/watch?v=eJbZHcB3mpE

More Life Health Seniors. (6 August 2018). Simple seated core strengthening workout for seniors. [Video]. https://www.youtube.com/watch?v=6Ts-deSDnRM

National Council on Aging. (22 October 2021). 5 tips to help older adults stay motivated to exercise. https://www.ncoa.org/article/5-tips-to-help-older-adults-stay-motivated-to-exercise

National Institute on Aging. (2022). How older adults can get started with exercise. *U.S. Department of Health & Human Services*. https://www.nia.nih.gov/health/how-older-adults-can-get-started-exercise

National Institute on Aging. (2022). Staying motivated to exercise: Tips for older adults. *U.S. Department of Health & Human Services*. https://www.nia.nih.gov/health/staying-motivated-exercise-tips-older-adults

Nina. (4 June 2021). Complete guide to workout clothes for women over 50. *Sharing a Journey*. https://sharingajourney.com/complete-guide-to-workout-clothes-for-women-over-50/

Olson, G. & Minnis, G. (5 October 2021). What is delayed onset muscle soreness (DOMS) and what can you do about it? *Healthline*. https://www.healthline.com/health/doms

Resnik, A., Bain, B., & Johnson, A. (13 October 2021). From reps to sets, your complete strength training glossary. *Byrdie*. https://www.byrdie.com/what-are-reps-sets-in-strength-training-5185170

Ricketts, D. & Shinn, J. (2022). The 3 principles of training: Overload, specificity, & progression. *Study.com*. https://study.com/academy/lesson/the-3-principles-of-training-overload-specificity-progression.html

Rizzo, N. (8 August 2021). 78 science backed benefits of weightlifting for seniors. *RunRepeat*. https://runrepeat.com/weightlifting-benefits-seniors

Rodriguez, D. (5 June 2018). Choosing the right workout clothes. *Everyday Health*. https://www.everydayhealth.com/fitness/choosing-workout-clothes.aspx

Ros, G. (2022). 3 day split workout - the complete guide. *HEVY*. https://www.hevyapp.com/3-day-split-workout-complete-guide/

Rogers, P. & Laferrara, T. (2 May 2022). Guide to sets, reps, and rest time in strength training. *VeryWell Fit.* https://www.verywellfit.com/beginners-guide-to-sets-repetitions-and-rest-intervals-3498619

Sarnataro, B. & DerSarkissian, C. (6 March 2022). Sore muscles? Don't stop exercising. *Jump Start.* https://www.webmd.com/fitness-exercise/features/sore-muscles-dont-stop-exercising

Scott, J. & Laferrara, T. (18 January 2021). How to start resistance training. *VeryWell Fit.* https://www.verywellfit.com/what-is-resistance-training-3496094

Seguin, R., Epping, J., Buchner, D., Bloch, R., & Nelson, M. (2002). Growing stronger: Strength training for older adults. *John Hancock Center for Physical Activity and Nutrition at the Friedman School of Nutrition Science and Policy at Tufts University.* https://www.cdc.gov/physicalactivity/downloads/growing_stronger.pdf

Seguin, R. & Nelson, M. (October 2003). The benefits of strength training for older adults. *American Journal of Preventive Medicine, 25*(3). pp. 141 - 149. https://doi.org/10.1016/S0749-3797(03)00177-6

Snug Safety. (9 June 2020). 5 core exercises for seniors: Build strength from your center. https://www.snugsafe.com/all-posts/core-exercises-for-seniors

Stelter, G. & Pletcher, P. (19 December 2017). 5 gentle back pain stretches for seniors. *Healthline.* https://www.healthline.com/health/back-pain/stretches-for-seniors

Tiley, C. (2018). What are reps and sets? *Never Too Old To Lift.* https://nevertoooldtolift.com/reps-and-sets/

Wikipedia. (6 January 2022). Morio Higaonna. https://en.wikipedia.org/wiki/Morio_Higaonna

Young, E. (16 December 2021). Work out at home: DIY Free Weights. *Family Handyman.* https://www.familyhandyman.com/article/diy-free-weights/

Printed in Great Britain
by Amazon

47770031R00145